Safer Sexy

attitude

Capital Gay

m*illivres ltd*

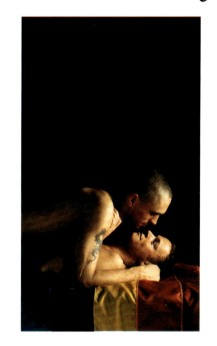

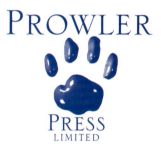

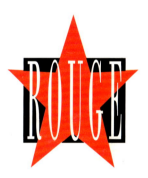

Sponsored by ivan massow associates

Sponsorship

Safer Sexy has been produced with the generous sponsorship of Ivan Massow Associates. Through the creation of the *Safer Sexy*/Ivan Massow HIV Prevention Fund, The Terrence Higgins Trust and Gay Men Fighting AIDS will receive donations from the sales of this book to help finance new safer sex education campaigns targetted at gay and bisexual men.

gay money → straight advice

ivan massow associates

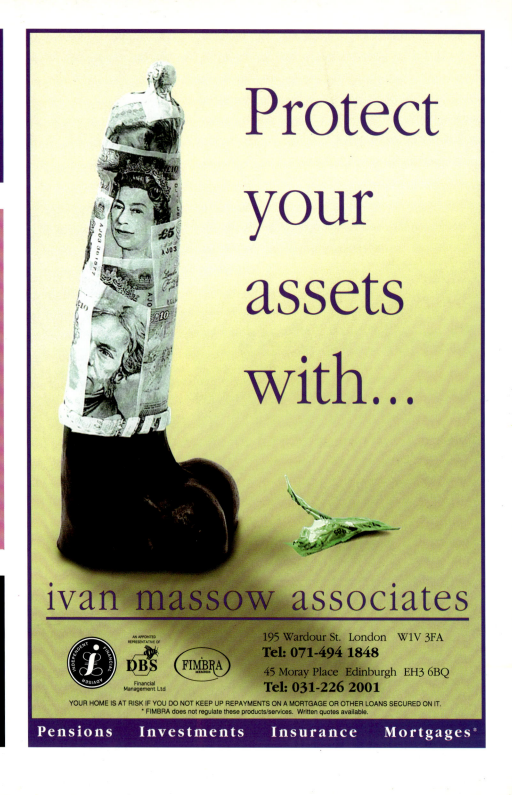

Safer Sexy

The guide to gay sex safely

Peter Tatchell

Photographs by Robert Taylor

FREEDOM EDITIONS

Dedication

Safer Sexy is dedicated to the memory of AIDS activists, Michael Callen and Jim Wilson, and in honour of lesbian, gay and bisexual people worldwide, who have done so much to promote safer sex and save the lives of millions. Evidence of the extraordinary contribution of queers to AIDS prevention is visible all around us in the lives of the living.

Legal Warning

Enjoy gay sex, but be careful. In Britain and some other countries gay orgies, cruising, backroom sex and SM causing injury are illegal.

Freedom Editions
(an imprint of the Cassell Group)
Villiers House
41-47 Strand
London
WC2N 5JE

387 Park Avenue South
New York
NY 10016-8810

© Peter Tatchell 1994

All rights reserved. No part of this publication may be reproduced or transmitted in any form or by any means, electronic or mechanical including photocopying, recording or any storage information or retrieval system, without prior permission in writing from the publishers.

First published 1994

British Library Cataloguing-in-Publication Data
A catalogue record for this book is available from the British Library.

ISBN 1 86047 000 9

Printed and bound in Great Britain

Peter Tatchell — Author and creative director

Peter Tatchell is one of Britain's leading activists for AIDS awareness and lesbian and gay equality.

He has written, lectured and campaigned for improved safer sex education, and for the human rights of people with HIV, since the beginning of the AIDS epidemic. His articles have appeared in *The Guardian*, *Sunday Times*, *Independent*, *Tribune*, *New Statesman*, *Time Out*, *Capital Gay*, *Pink Paper* and *Gay Times*.

From the mid-1980's Peter Tatchell helped draft local authority AIDS strategies and Labour Party policy statements on AIDS. He was also one of the earliest advocates of the European Community Programme Against AIDS.

His pioneering self-help book, *AIDS: A Guide to Survival*, published in 1986, broke new ground in offering hope where others counselled only fear and fatalism. Its defiant, fightback approach has since helped many thousands of people with AIDS live longer and better quality lives.

In 1987, Peter Tatchell founded the UK AIDS Vigil Organisation – the first movement set up in Britain to defend the civil liberties of people with HIV – and drafted the world's first comprehensive 'AIDS & Human Rights Charter' to challenge the escalating trend towards government repression.

The following year, he coordinated a massive candlelit procession in London, which resulted in the World Health Ministers' Summit on AIDS amending its final declaration to include a specific commitment to oppose AIDS-related discrimination. This commitment marked a turning point in the attitude of many governments, from panic and suppression to education and support.

One of the founder members of the London ACT UP (the AIDS Coalition To Unleash Power) in 1989, and of the lesbian and gay direct action group OutRage! in 1990, Peter Tatchell has campaigned for mandatory sex education in all primary and secondary schools, including explicit and non-judgemental information about homosexuality and AIDS prevention. This campaign has involved the leafletting of school students to combat the censorship of information about HIV and lesbian and gay sexuality.

Peter Tatchell is also the author of *Europe In The Pink: Lesbian & Gay Equality In The New Europe* (GMP London 1992). In 1995, Cassell will publish his new book, *Fighting Back Against HIV: Self-Help for the Newly Diagnosed*.

Robert Taylor — Photographer

Robert Taylor is a freelance photographer whose pictures range from intimate portraiture, through to public relations and erotic imagery.

His photographs have been exhibited in London, Paris, Arles, New York and Los Angeles.

As well as working in educational publishing in Europe and West Africa, specializing in sex education, Robert Taylor's photographs have featured in safer sex campaigns for local authorities and AIDS organisations.

Contents

Acknowledgements 6

Preface 7

Pride and Passion 9

Saving lives and living well Love rights **In praise of difference** It's a queer world **Pride and defiance**

Safer Sexy Attitude 13

Rethinking sex A positive alternative **Negotiating safer sex** Practice makes perfect **Saying no – hearing no**

Sexy Without Risk 18

Protection for us all Assessing the risks **HIV safer sex checklist**

Turning on to rubber 24

Cum in a condom Be prepared **Which is safest?** Varieties and styles **Lubrication** Spermicides **Protecting condoms** Condom sense **Putting it on and taking it off** Latex barriers

Sex Satisfaction 30

Communicating desires Observation and imitation **Sameness or difference?** Reciprocation **Diversity** Inventiveness **Avoidance of routine** Versatility **Danger-free**

Down to Passion 32

Erogenous zones Kissing **Food** Love-bites **Caressing** Massage **Fingering** Licking arse **Tit play** Noise **Sex toys** Fantasy **Explore and excite**

Cumming Together 42

Good orgasms Jerking off **Rubbing bodies** Sucking dick **Fucking arse**

Diversity and Spice 59

Love and let love Fetishes and fixations **Threesomes and orgies** Dirty sex **Anonymous quickies** Porn **Sex over the phone** Watching and showing off **Piercing** Shaving **Piss** Shit **Fisting** Sadomasochism **Bondage** Pain pleasure

Sex Problems and Solutions 75

Cumming too fast Inability to cum **Lack of erection** Sex compulsion **Drug or alcohol dependence**

Cruising Safely 81

Making contact Checking him over **Coping with rejection** Cruisewise safety **Safe pick ups** Avoiding arrest

One Man or Many? 87

Needs and choices Settling down **Playing the field**

Love and Relationships 90

Formulas for success Open or closed relationships **Dealing with difficulties** Breaking up

Looking After Yourself 98

Safety first Getting fresh **Turn-offs and remedies** Healthy queer

The HIV test 104

To test or not?

Preventable Diseases & Conditions 108

AIDS Amoebiasis **Cancers** Chancroid **Chlamydia** Crabs **Cystitis** Glandular fever **Gonorrhoea** Gut infections **Hepatitis** Herpes **HIV** Molluscum contagiosum **Non-specific urethritis and proctitis** Prostatitis **Scabies** Syphilis **Trichomoniasis** Warts **The ABC of prevention**

Acknowledgements

My thanks to Professor Anthony Pinching of the Medical College of Saint Bartholomew's Hospital, Dr Brian Gazzard and Dr Mike Youle of Chelsea and Westminster Hospital, John Howson of Camden and Islington Health Advisors Team, Simon Watney of the Red Hot AIDS Charitable Trust, Derek Cohen of SM Gays and particuarly to Edward King of the National AIDS Manual, for their valuable advice concerning the text.

My gratitude to my publisher, Steve Cook, for his support and courage in producing such a groundbreaking book; and to Ben Cracknell for his superb design work.

My special appreciation to Robert Taylor, the photographer, for his creative collaboration in interpreting my ideas to produce such striking images.

Last, but not least, my thanks to Expectations for the sex toys and fetish gear, and to the models: Danny Cooper, Mikki Farrar, Daniel Frost, Farouk Gohil, Darren Hartley, Rey Hernandez, Jason Muir, David Porter, Edward Pritchett, Nathan Reid, Errol Sanquez, Nathan Seamer, TN Tran, and Geoff Whittaker.

I owe much of my inspiration for this book to the heroes and heroines of OutRage!, ACT UP, Queer Nation and Gay Men Fighting AIDS whose sacrifice, imagination, determination and courage have contributed so much to awareness and action against HIV, and to the struggle for the dignity, self-determination and human rights of lesbian, gay and bisexual people.

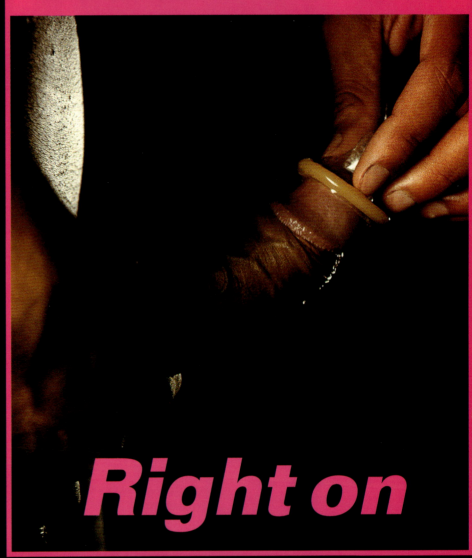

Hard on Rubber on Right on

Preface

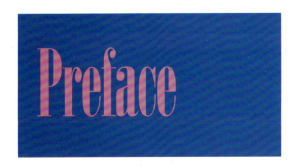

Safer Sexy is a valuable and innovative contribution to the fight against AIDS. The first truly comprehensive guide to safer gay sex between men, it draws on the lessons of earlier successful HIV prevention campaigns which have shown that the most effective way to encourage the adoption of safer sex is by using sexy images which glamourize risk reduction and by using explicit language which makes the facts accessible to everyone.

Breaking new ground in sex education and AIDS awareness, this book recognizes that the promotion of gay self-esteem and self-empowerment is a crucial aspect of the fight against HIV. By encouraging gay and bisexual men to feel worthwhile, confident and proud, *Safer Sexy* also encourages them to take care of themselves and their friends.

Its gay-positive message is to live life well without putting yourself, or your partners, at risk of HIV and other sexually-transmitted diseases. This is a thoroughly moral message which emphasizes that sex should always by safe, consenting and mutually fulfilling.

The more people who read this book and follow its advice, the sooner the AIDS epidemic will be halted. We are happy to endorse the empowering, life-saving message of *Safer Sexy*:

Dr David Bradford
Australian National Council on AIDS;
Vice President of the Australasian College of Venereologists

Clint George
Sexual Health Officer, Black HIV/AIDS Network

Robin Gorna
AIDS activist and worker, specializing in women and bisexuality; Head of Lobbying of the European AIDS Treatment Group

Jonathan Grimshaw
Co-Founder, Body Positive and The Landmark; Chair, National AIDS Manual

Ceri Hutton
Director, Immunity

Shivananda Khan
Chief Executive, The NAZ Project

Edward King
Editor, *AIDS Treatment Update*; Co-Director, Gay Men Fighting AIDS

Nick Partridge
Chief Executive, The Terrence Higgins Trust

Professor Anthony Pinching
Professor of Immunology, Medical College of St. Bartholomew's Hospital, London

Trisha Plummer
Director, Blackliners

Peter Scott
Chair, Gay Men Fighting AIDS; Founding Editor, National AIDS Manual

Dr Joseph Sonnabend
Medical Director, Community Research Initiative On AIDS, New York

Christopher Spence
Director, London Lighthouse

Simon Watney
Director, Red Hot AIDS Charitable Trust

Professor Jonathan Weber
Professor of GU Medicine, St. Mary's Hospital Medical School, London

Dr Ian Williams
Senior Lecturer GU Medicine, University College Medical School, London

Phill Wilson
Director of Public Policy, AIDS Project Los Angeles

Dr Mike Youle
HIV & AIDS Trials Coordinator, Chelsea and Westminster Hospital, London

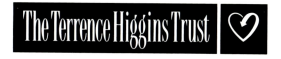

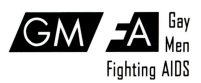

'*Safer Sexy* empowers young people who are coming out so they can have more control over their lives and prevent HIV'   BOY GEORGE

'If only there had been a book like this in the early 1980s when the AIDS epidemic began, perhaps fewer gay men would have become infected. This book will save lives'   HOLLY JOHNSON

'Erotic, comprehensive and common-sensical; *Safer Sexy* is aimed at those who most need to read it. Let's hope they do.'   SIR IAN MCKELLEN

'No horny bugger's sex life will be complete without this saucy accessory.'   JIMMY SOMERVILLE

SAFER SEX
LOVE LIFE

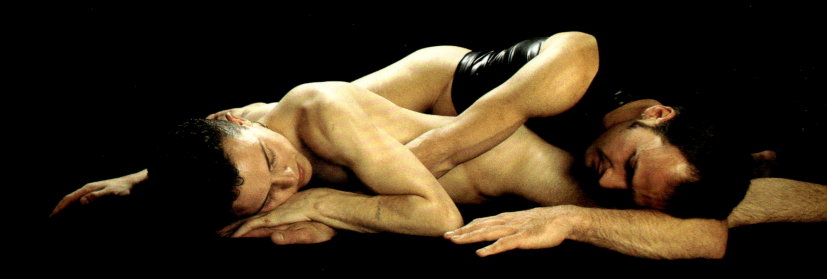

Pride and Passion
Love rights

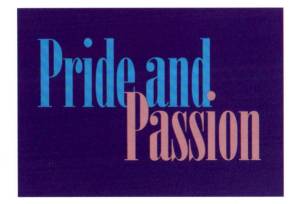

Saving lives and living well

Safer Sexy is about saving lives and living life well. Homophobia and censorship are killing gay and bisexual men by preventing us from getting straightforward and sexy information about how to have gay sex safely.

Safer Sexy confronts this neglect by presenting the facts about disease prevention in a way that is explicit, educative, erotic, entertaining and empowering. Its life-saving theme is that good sex doesn't have to be dangerous, and that safer sex can be great sex. This upbeat message applies equally to guys who are HIV positive and HIV negative, and to those who don't know their HIV status.

Safer Sexy is also about the validation and celebration of queer desire and sexual diversity. Prejudice and guilt are causing psychological and emotional harm to many gay and bisexual men.

Safer Sexy counteracts this damage by promoting gay self-esteem, sexual satisfaction and emotional fulfilment; it offers a sex-positive and homo-affirmative guide to gay love and lust without risk.

NOWADAYS IT'S COOL TO BE QUEER

Love rights

The right to love a person of the same sex, and to enjoy a happy and healthy sex life, is a fundamental human right. Yet governments and religions worldwide conspire to sustain sexual ignorance, guilt, prejudice and ill-health. The homophobia they encourage is responsible for erotic and emotional misery on a massive scale. It is also contributing to the needless spread of HIV infection because many gay and bisexual men, especially teenagers, are being denied adequate information about safer sex.

Cool queers cum in condoms

The world does not have to be like this. Sex is not dirty. The human body is not obscene. Gay sexuality is not immoral. Homophobia is not natural. AIDS is not inevitable. We all have a right to sexual self-determination. We all have a right to love the person of our choice. We all have a right to sexual health and happiness. It is up to you to claim your right to be gay and to live your life with pride, dignity and fulfilment. It is within your power to protect yourself and those you love against HIV and other preventable diseases.

You can help change the world. Begin with your own life. Come out. Stand up for queer rights. Practise safer sex. Love people with AIDS. Support the lesbian and gay community. Encourage your friends to do likewise. Together, we can defeat homophobia and HIV.

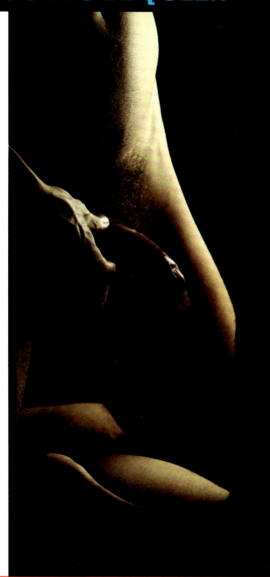

Are You A Cool Condom Queer?

Suck a fruit
flavoured condom

In praise of difference

To be human is to be sexual. A world without sexuality is unthinkable, and impossible. Queer sex is part of the wonderful diversity of human sexuality. This sexual difference, like cultural and ethnic differences, enlivens and enriches our whole society.

Gay relationships and lifestyles are often very different from those of the average heterosexual. They encompass notions and experiences that many straights could learn from. As the sex researchers William Masters and Virginia Johnson documented in *Homosexuality In Perspective*, queers tend to be more sexually adventurous. We have a wider repertoire of sexual acts, and experience a higher level of erotic satisfaction. Compared to most straights, our relationships are usually more equal, and we are more experimental when it comes to partnership patterns. We don't need a marriage certificate to validate our love and, more recently, it is gay men who have pioneered safer sex and adapted best to safer sex practice. The fact that homosexuals are different from heterosexuals is a positive virtue and a reason for pride.

Sucking is low risk. But if you want to be super-safe use a condom

It's a queer world

Lesbians and gay men are everywhere. We're in every country and every culture on our planet. Despite all attempts at repression, including the Nazi policy of mass extermination, we just keep bouncing back. Irrepressible! Irresistible!

Recent sex surveys in Britain, France and the United States suggesting a very low incidence of homosexuality have been methodologically flawed. Their random sampling technique failed to take into account the concentration of gay men in large cities, and interviewing people in their own homes made closeted homosexuals reluctant to reveal themselves, especially if they lived with their families and feared exposure.

Studies in the United States during the 1940s by the sexologist Dr Alfred Kinsey are also imperfect and may slightly over-estimate the incidence of same-sex relations. Nevertheless, they remain the most authoritative research on the subject. Kinsey's findings, *Sexual Behaviour In The Human Male*, suggest that about 10% of the male population is mainly or exclusively gay. A further 15% is mostly heterosexual but homosexual occasionally. Altogether, over a third of men have gay sex at least once during their lifetime, and roughly half have some experience of emotional or sexual feeling towards other men (sometimes transitory and unexpressed).

Even if queer desire was only half as common as Kinsey recorded, that would still be quite extraordinary given the immense social pressures to be straight. It stands to reason that gayness would probably be much more widespread in a homo-positive culture.

Most guys, it seems, are born with the potential to be gay. There may be biological factors which influence sexual orientation. But psychological and anthropological evidence indicates that social factors are more significant.

The psychoanalytic investigations of Sigmund Freud led him to conclude, in *Three Essays On Sexuality* and *An Autobiographical Study*, that everyone is born constitutionally bisexual, with a homosexual capability. Our erotic desires are initially pluralistic and diverse, without any differentiation between hetero and homo attraction. Sexual orientation evolves during childhood through a complex developmental process which is influenced by personal experience, particularly within the family. The implication is that homosexuality and heterosexuality are, in the main, socially determined rather than being biologically innate.

This view is reinforced by the research of the anthropologists Clellan Ford and Frank Beach. In *Patterns Of Sexual Behaviour* they recorded details of some tribal cultures in which all young men go through a period of homosexuality as part of their rites of passage into manhood. Once completed, the majority become heterosexual. If sexuality was biologically predetermined, these men would never be able to switch from heterosexuality to homosexuality, and then back again, with such apparent ease. This suggests that the decisive factors influencing sexual orientation are social expectations and cultural values.

Since nearly everyone is potentially queer, access to gay safer sex advice is everyone's right, and the struggle for queer human rights is in everyone's interest. Queer liberation is about the right of everyone to experience the joys of gay desire without guilt, discrimination, or the risk of HIV.

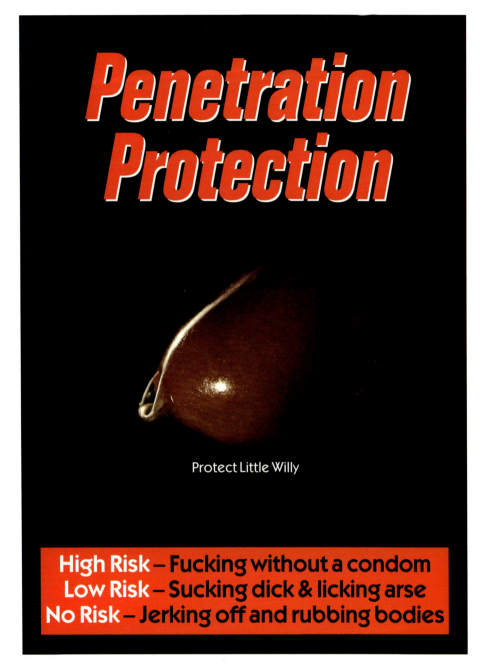

Pride and Passion
It's a queer world

Penetration Protection

Protect Little Willy

High Risk – Fucking without a condom
Low Risk – Sucking dick & licking arse
No Risk – Jerking off and rubbing bodies

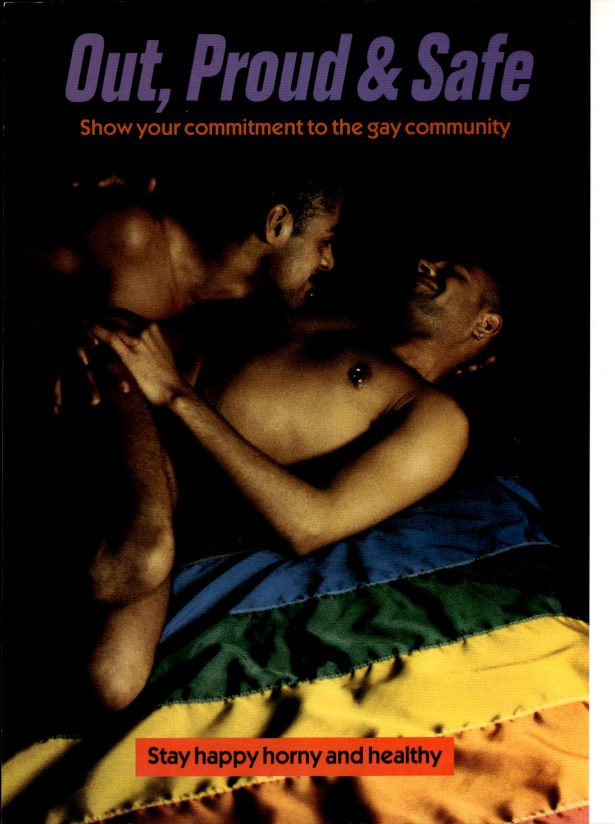

Out, Proud & Safe
Show your commitment to the gay community

Stay happy horny and healthy

Pride and defiance

The concept of safer sex was invented by gay men to protect ourselves and our community from HIV. It has led to the most rapid and successful health-enhancing changes in sexual behaviour in human history. We queers have done it for ourselves, and saved thousands of lives. We can all be proud of that. Straights could learn from us.

The safer sex revolution is a remarkable achievement which we need to sustain, both for our own sake as individual gay men and for the sake of all gay men collectively. Shamefully, many health and education authorities do not target HIV prevention education at gay and bisexual men. Those that do often censor the safer sex message to appease homophobes. When straight society ignores our health needs in this way, we have to respond by looking after ourselves. That means adopting safer sex, and encouraging our lovers and friends to do likewise.

As the whole history of the lesbian and gay community has taught us, we can never rely on heterosexuals to help us. We can only depend on each other and our own self-help energies. Already, HIV has claimed far too many people, including artists, writers, activists, volunteers and many others who have made their own contribution to queer freedom by living their lives with pride and dignity. Their loss diminishes the lesbian and gay community, indeed our whole society. The best way we can honour their memory, and the courage of people currently living with AIDS, is by making sure we don't give or get the virus.

Practising safer sex is an act of queer pride and defiance. It is our refusal to allow HIV to destroy our community and its achievements. It is our affirmation that gay is good and that queers deserve to love without fear. It is a statement that we care about each other and our futures.

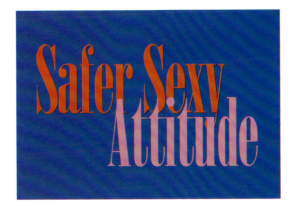

Safer Sexy Attitude

Rethinking sex

Safer sex is pro-sex. Real sex. Sexy sex. Raunchy without risk, it's about having sex in ways that are satisfying and safe. Far from being less sexy or a chore, safer sex is simply a different, risk-free way of experiencing sexual pleasure. What safer sex involves is redirecting our sexual desire, not denying or diminishing it. To avoid the danger of HIV, we need to make some adjustments in our erotic techniques. But it is still possible to have horny passion and fantastic orgasms. The end result is good sex in new ways which keep us and our partners safe.

Safer sex is a sexual revolution. Rethinking our attitudes towards sex, it offers new ideas on the nature of sexual satisfaction, and the means by which erotic ecstasy is achieved. The main obstacle to playing safely is sexual conservatism and conditioning. The traditional assumption is that sex is all, or mainly, about fucking. Everything else is seen as mere kids' stuff or foreplay. Safer sex challenges this assumption. It rejects the idea that fucking is the be-all and end-all of sexual satisfaction. Instead, it suggests there are many different, and equally satisfying, routes to a great orgasm.

Of course, fucking is fun. But screwing is not essential for sexual fulfilment. What is important is

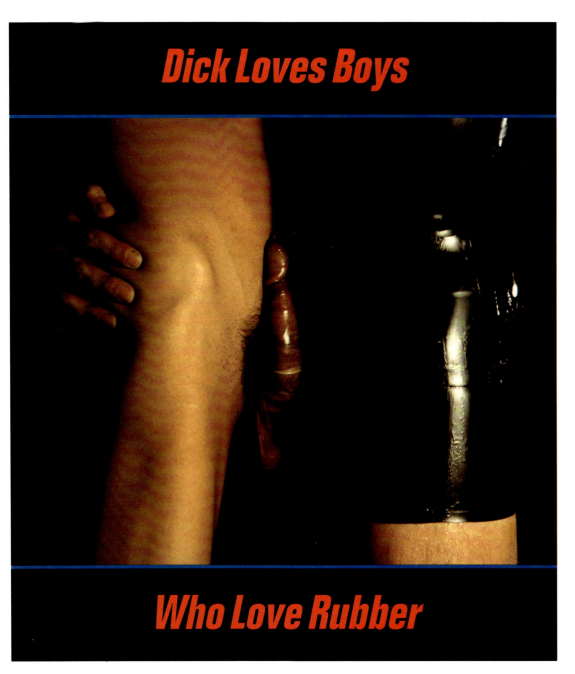

Dick Loves Boys

Who Love Rubber

Safer Sexy Attitude | Safer Sexy

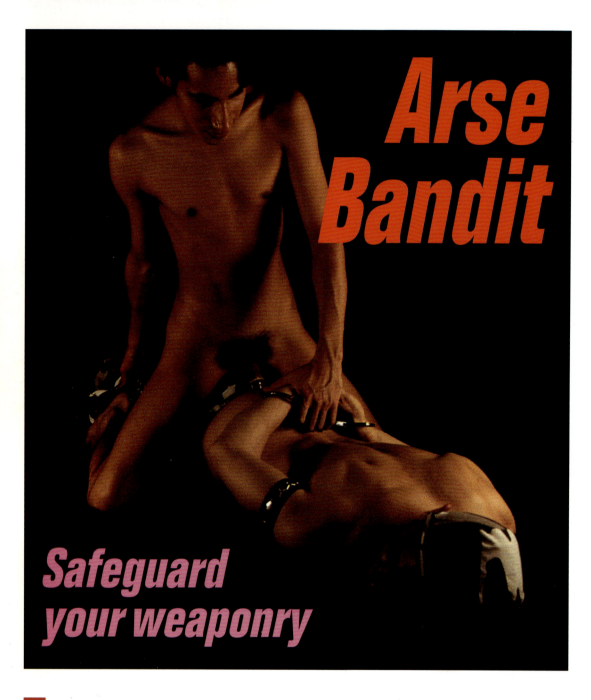

Arse Bandit

Safeguard your weaponry

not the method of orgasm, but the quality of orgasm. It is possible to have a fabulous, frenzied sexual climax without fucking. All it takes is a little imagination and practice.

One of the great virtues of safer sex is that it encourages us to think about what we do in bed. It opens up new erotic possibilities. Instead of sex by rote – a predictable routine which so often revolves around fucking – safer sex puts renewed emphasis on those immensely pleasurable dimensions of sex that are frequently skated over in the rush to screw. Safer sex expands our erotic horizons and spices our sexual experiences with new delights – the multitude of erogenous zones, the diverse methods of erotic stimulation, and the sensation-heightening power of sex toys and fantasy.

In contrast to social expectation and pressure, safer sex validates the right not to fuck and the right to choose non-fucking alternatives. It is about sexual choice and diversity. The human species has an extraordinary capacity for rational thought and creative behaviour. Our ability to reflect, reason and re-evaluate, means that we are able to question the assumption that sex is just about fucking. It gives us the power to experiment sexually and to innovate.

Safer sex is a creative development in human sexuality. It is about using our imagination to have good sex in new ways which protect ourselves and the men we love to love.

A positive alternative

This positive view of safer sex is crucial to its success. If you feel negative, and think safer sex will be boring and unsatisfying, then it probably will be. As with everything, a person's expectations affect the outcome. A negative attitude tends to produce a negative experience, whereas a positive feeling is likely to produce a positive result.

We therefore need to see safer sex not just as a lifesaver and health-promoter. It is also a way of taking the fear and anxiety out of sex, of creating diversity in our range of erotic experiences. Looked at positively, safer sex is a great plus for our sexual and emotional experiences.

Another positive way of viewing safer sex is as a challenge, not as a defeat or frustration. Sure, there are some forms of sex that are no longer safe, but it is not too difficult to find new forms of risk-free passion. The need to avoid danger is simply a challenge to our sense of sexual adventure and inventiveness. All it requires is a new mindset willing to explore the many exciting, safe ways we can rub flesh and shoot cum.

Still, some guys find it difficult to adapt. Those of us who feel uncomfortable and unsatisfied initially about playing safely should remember that much of what we enjoy about sex involves overcoming inhibitions. At first, some men find sucking cock and fucking arse a complete turn-off. Yet over time, they come to like the idea, and these forms of sex often become favourite activities.

In the same way, successful, enjoyable safer sex means opening our minds to new erotic possibilities and having a positive attitude towards them.

Negotiating safer sex

One of the big advantages of safer sex is that it encourages communication between us about what we feel safe doing, and about what kinds of sex we enjoy. This results in greater intimacy and sharing. So how do we negotiate safer sex with a partner?

It can work non-verbally simply by physically steering a guy's body away from attempts at risky practices towards those that are risk-free. If he tries to thrust inside your arse without a condom, for example, swing your body around and take his dick inside

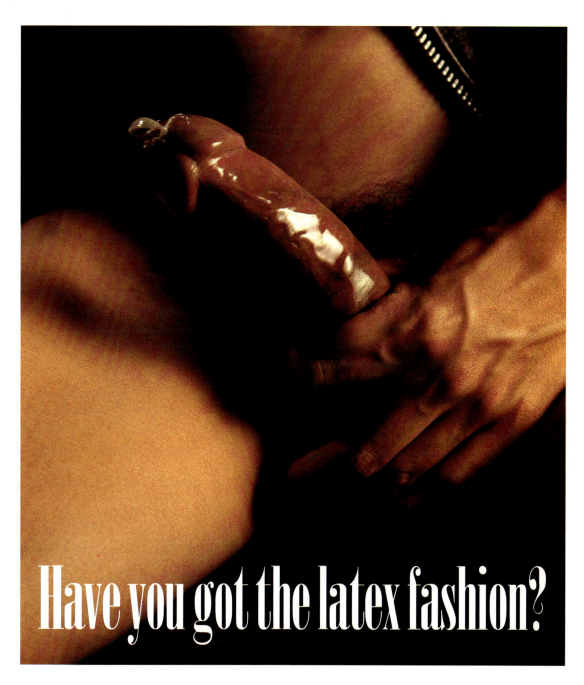

Have you got the latex fashion?

Men Who Love Men Love to Protect Them

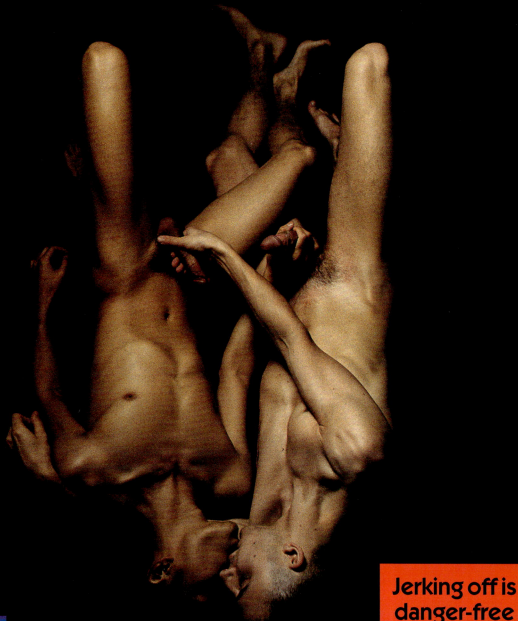

Jerking off is danger-free

your mouth. Slide your lips up and down his shaft. Tickle the head of his cock with your tongue. This will often give him so much delight that his desire to fuck will wane and he will probably be quite happy for you to suck him off instead. If he still insists on screwing, roll a condom down his dick with your mouth. Presto! You are ready for safe fucking.

The best way to avoid any misunderstandings, and ensure that safer sex goes smoothly and is mutually satisfying, is by talking to your partner soon after you start kissing and touching, and before you get as far as clothes on the floor.

For some guys this is embarrassing. You may feel awkward talking about safer sex. Yet your partner often has the same inhibitions. Someone has to take the plunge! Don't worry if you fumble a bit with shyness. It can be quite endearing and sympathy-evoking. Most of us appreciate a man who is smart, and who is concerned enough to think about our well-being as well as his own. You can also signal your commitment to safer sex to a new partner by having a jar of condoms next to your bed or a safer sex poster on your wall.

Practice makes perfect

Great sex is a matter of experience and practice. Being good in bed (or in the bushes) is an acquired skill. Taking a dick right down your throat, for example, is not easy at first. To overcome the gagging sensation is quite an art. However, once you've mastered the technique, deep-throating is fabulous.

Safer sex is no different. It involves learning new sensual techniques. A little perseverance is required. As with anything new, safer sex rarely goes right to begin with. It has to be practised and perfected. Most of us mess up the first few times we use a condom. We roll it on the wrong way, or fail to smooth out the wrinkles. Some of us lose our hard-on. When we try alternatives to fucking, such as jerking off or rubbing bodies together, we sometimes find it difficult initially to have a good orgasm. So what's new? We've all been through those difficulties and most of us have overcome them. Whichever way we have sex, it takes repeated experimentation and practice to get it right. The same is true of safer sex. Over time, it becomes natural and instinctive. We do it almost automatically. Because it's safe, we feel relaxed and secure about sex. Without worries, we are free to concentrate on having fun. That's a wonderful liberating feeling.

A tip about condoms: if you find using them difficult, practice on yourself. Put on a rubber when you jerk off. It will help you get accustomed to using condoms – and enjoying them.

Saying no – hearing no

Each of us has the right to ask. Each of us has the right to refuse. Just because we go to bed with a man doesn't mean we are under an obligation to do whatever he demands.

If you don't enjoy certain activities, like being fucked or tied up, don't feel you have to do them. It's your right to control your own body. Never be afraid or embarrassed to ask a guy to stop when you don't like what he is doing. If he respects you, he will understand and accept your decision. Agreeing to sexual acts that you are not happy with, especially if they are unsafe, is not a sign of your commitment to another man. It is a sign that you are allowing yourself to be manipulated and abused.

Some men use emotional blackmail to pressure their partners into unsafe sex. They claim that fucking without a condom is a test of commitment and trust. Bullshit! It's proof of selfishness and stupidity!

Aiming to please another guy is fine, even commendable. However, it is not okay if it means doing things which make you feel uncomfortable or which put you (or him) at risk of HIV.

Good sex is about negotiating what you want to do with your partner. It involves mutual agreement about what you both enjoy doing, and about what you both feel is safe. When you choose the kind of sex that is mutually secure and pleasurable, it makes for the best orgasms – and demonstrates genuine friendship and respect.

Sex is not compulsory. There is no obligation to have sex at all, with anyone, if you don't feel like it. Choosing to abstain totally from sex is a valid option. You may make this choice because you are distressed by the painful break up of a much valued relationship, or because you want to concentrate all your energies on an important and satisfying work project. Being free from the pressure to be sexually desirable and available can be a great relief, as can freedom from the emotional traumas of falling in and out of love. Abstaining from sex may enable you to become more aware of your non-sexual talents and friendships, which you may not have fully appreciated in the past. It can be an impetus to develop previously neglected aspects of your personality, such as creativity, humour and supportiveness. These attributes and skills are very worthwhile and can sometimes give just as much satisfaction as sex and relationships.

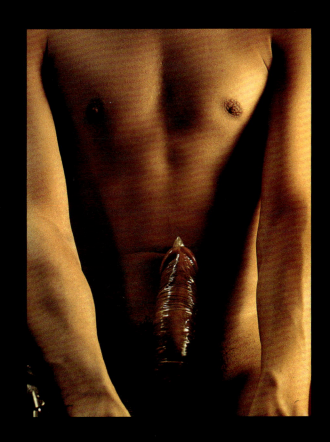

Condom Couture

For Buttfuckers with Style

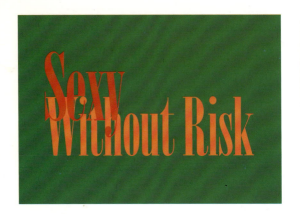

Protection for us all

Any of us can get HIV if we don't take precautions. Some of us already have the virus. Whatever our status, we can all protect ourselves and our partners against infection by practising safer sex.

Safer sex does not mean no sex or worse sex. It doesn't even mean clean sex. It means having good sex in fun ways which prevent the exchange of HIV. We can pick up the virus through either a one-night stand or a monogamous relationship. Being in love is no protection. Equally, promiscuity is not necessarily dangerous. The key to preventing HIV is not having fewer partners, but avoiding all risky behaviour. Guys who always practise safer sex can have lots of sex with lots of different partners without giving or getting HIV. However, those who have unsafe sex with their one and only partner run a very high risk of contracting HIV if that partner is already infected or becomes infected.

HIV affects men of all ages. You don't have to be old, or on the gay scene for a long time, to get the virus. Plenty of young guys are HIV positive. Likewise, HIV is not limited to people from particular social groups. It doesn't discriminate between the rubber fetishists and vanilla queens, between black

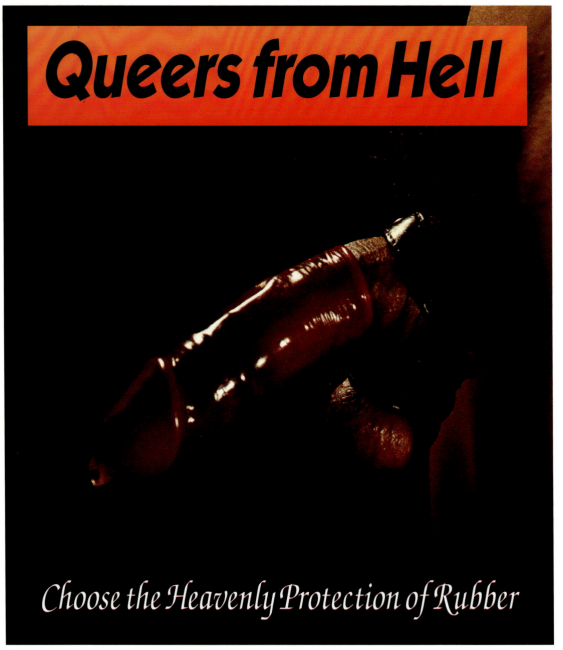

Sexy Without Risk
Protection for us all

and white, or rich and poor. Any gay or bisexual man who has unsafe sex anywhere is putting himself at risk.

Many guys have HIV without knowing it. You can't tell if a man has the virus by looking at him. Most guys with HIV look and feel healthy. They play sport, work-out at the gym, party all night. Some are, or have been, in longterm relationships. Indeed many gay men with HIV got it from a regular boyfriend who was not aware he had the virus. Since there is no way of knowing who has got HIV and who has not, it is best to assume that every partner you have may be infected. Stick to safer sex with everyone. That way, it doesn't matter if one of you has HIV. Safer sex will protect you both, always.

If your partner confides that he has HIV, there is no need to stop having sex with him. Just avoid risky behaviour. That way, there is no danger you'll get infected.

For guys who already have the virus, it is important to follow the safer sex guidelines to protect against additional exposure to HIV and other infectious diseases that might aggravate damage to the immune system and provoke serious illness. Repeated infection with HIV, especially with more aggressive strains of the virus, and even infection with less dangerous diseases such as hepatitis or gonorrhoea, could further weaken your immune defenses and hasten the onset of AIDS.

Suck Fuck Wank Spank

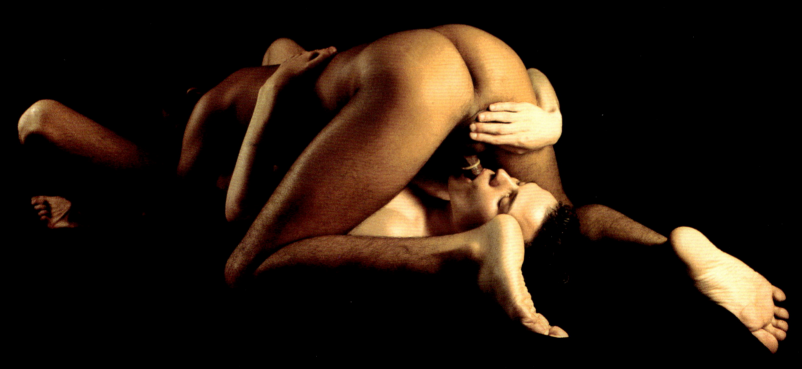

Safely

Sexy Without Risk / Safer Sexy

Assessing the risks

Some guys get the risks of various sexual acts out of proportion. They fuss about obscure or hypothetical routes of HIV transmission. They worry endlessly about whether they have cuts in their mouth or on their hands, and whether any cum got into these cuts when they were sucking or jerking off. It could be possible to get HIV in these ways, but it is very unlikely. You would have to be extremely unlucky. Very, very few people anywhere in the world have got HIV by these means.

While it's smart to take sensible safer sex precautions, there is no justification for being fanatical and obsessive. The priority is to avoid sexual activities that carry major risks, such as unprotected screwing, not total risk elimination. Sex would be boring and tedious if we tried to eliminate every single conceivable risk of giving or getting HIV. Indeed, the only absolutely guaranteed safe sex is no sex. That's not a realistic or necessary choice. It's obvious that some forms of sexual behaviour are much more risky than others. It's these high-risk acts, like being fucked without a condom, that we should concentrate on avoiding.

HIV is found in highly infectious amounts in blood and cum. Therefore, the key rule of safer sex is: don't let your partner get his blood or cum inside your body, and don't let your blood or cum get inside his body. HIV is also found in pre-cum. This is the sticky fluid that your dick produces in the early stages of sexual excitement before you cum. It's also infectious and should not be transferred from one body into another.

Serum is also rich in HIV. This is the clear liquid that exudes from the skin when it is squeezed, beaten or grazed. But you will probably not be exposed to it during sex unless you are involved in SM activities such as caning or tit torture.

Other body fluids can also contain HIV, albeit in minuscule amounts which are insufficient to be infectious. The only possible exception is the moisture and mucus found inside the arse, which may carry a small risk of infection. The risk increases significantly if arse juices get blood in them, as sometimes happens during fucking, fingering and fisting.

Spit, piss and shit cannot normally transmit HIV, but they can become infectious if they are contaminated with blood from an internal wound or infection. Tears and sweat are no danger at all.

Non-penetrative sex, such as jerking off and rubbing bodies, is safest. If you don't put bits of your body (especially your cock) into your partner's body, or vice versa, there is virtually no chance of body fluids which may be infectious passing from one guy to another. HIV cannot pass through healthy, undamaged skin. If you haven't got any open cuts or skin rashes, it is absolutely safe for your partner to shoot his cum over your body.

So far as penetrative sex is concerned, fucking without a rubber is infinitely more risky than prick-sucking and arse-kissing.

More information about degrees of risk associated with particular sexual acts are in the chapters 'Down to Passion', 'Cumming Together' and 'Diversity and Spice'. In the meantime, here's a brief guide to what is safe and what is low-risk for HIV.

Kissing is very safe. The only very rare danger of HIV infection arises in the extremely unlikely coincidence that both you and your partner have open wounds and bleeding in your mouths or on your lips.

Jerking off and rubbing bodies are also very safe, but cover any cuts or sores with a waterproof sticking plaster.

Sucking dick is low-risk, so long as your mouth is healthy and undamaged. If you want to be extra safe, get him to pull his dick out of your mouth before he cums. Whenever there are sores or bleeding in your mouth, or on his dick, make sure he puts on a condom before you suck him.

Fucking arse with a condom is safe, providing you use a strong condom, plenty of water-based lube (not spit, cum or oil-based creams), and check regularly to make sure the condom has not broken or slipped off.

Thigh and butt rubbing are extra safe because they don't involve penetration.

Licking arse is very low-risk for HIV. However, if he hasn't showered, or if you want to lick inside his butt, use a latex barrier to avoid other infections such as hepatitis.

Fingering and fisting arse are safe unless you damage the inside of his butt or have open wounds on your fingers, hands or arms (in which case, wear rubber gloves). However, it is risky to interchange fingers or hands between your partner's arse and your own arse.

Many gay and bisexual men also have sex with women. With rising levels of HIV transmission during straight sex, it is important to protect you and your female partner. Always use a condom for fucking.

No form of safer sex is 100% safe. Condoms break occasionally. However, safer sex can reduce the risk of HIV to negligible proportions. Different sexual activities involve different levels of risk. Some of these risks – especially concerning kissing, sucking, licking and fingering – are mainly theoretical. They need a set of exceptional circumstances, and rare coincidences like an open cut that gets soaked in cum, to put us in danger. Studies of thousands of gay men worldwide have shown that screwing without a condom is responsible for nearly all cases of HIV infection. Only a tiny minority have got HIV from any other sexual activity. If cock-sucking or arse-licking could pass on the virus easily, a lot more of us would be infected, and research would have revealed this by now.

It is up to each of us to consider the various degrees of risk and make our own choice about how much risk we are prepared to take when having sex. Some guys prefer the security of no-risk. Others find that too restrictive and decide that low-risk activities are acceptable. What is important to remember is that of all gay sex acts, fucking without a condom is by far the easiest way to transmit HIV. It is much more risky than sucking or any other form of sex. Avoiding unprotected fucking is therefore our number one priority. Using a condom when you screw is the single most important safer sex commitment you can ever make.

Healthy tips

♂ Showering before and after sex is good personal hygiene and can get rid of germs like hepatitis from around your arse-hole, which makes it safer to lick.

♂ Never share sex toys such like vibrators, dildoes and butt plugs; this could transfer infection from him to you (and vice versa).

♂ Pissing straight after sex clears the dick-hole of cum. This stops you dribbling and spreading spunk around. After using a condom with spermicide, it also gets rid of any irritating chemical residues from inside your cock.

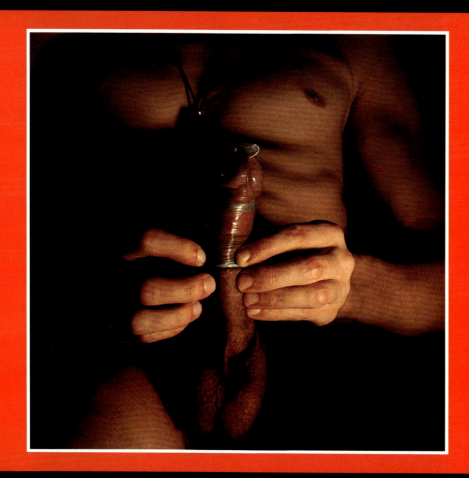

Sexy Without Risk
Assessing the risks

If he hasn't got it on

Don't let him get it off

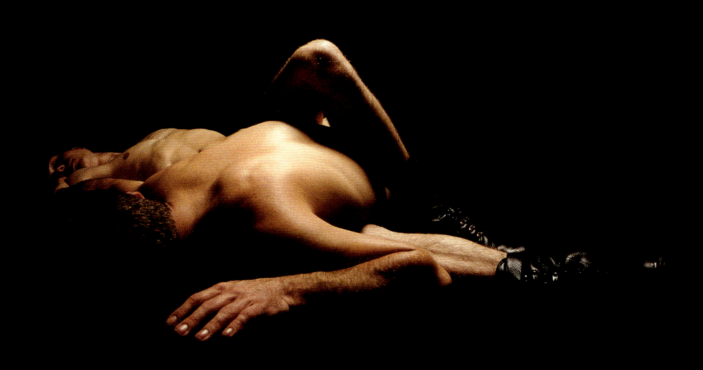

HIV Safer sex checklist

> Very high risk – Screwing without a condom.
>
> Low risk – Cock-sucking and licking arse.
>
> No risk – Rubbing bodies and jerking off.

Safest sex

- Kissing and caressing.

- Licking nipples, balls, shaft of the dick, and outside of the arse-hole.

- Cumming without penetration: jerking off and rubbing bodies.

Safer sex

- Fucking arse with a condom.

- Sucking dick, providing there are no cuts in the mouth or on the cock (if there are, suck with a condom).

- Licking inside the arse using a latex barrier.

- Fingering and fisting the arse, as long as there is no internal bleeding and the skin on the finger, hand or arm is undamaged (otherwise use rubber gloves).

- Pissing and shitting which does not enter the body.

- Biting and whipping that avoids breaking the skin.

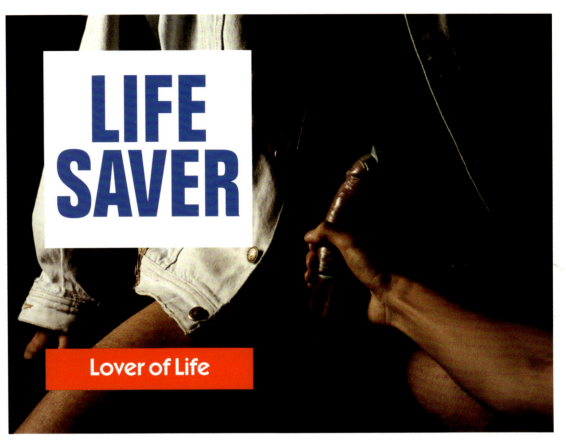

Unsafe sex

- Licking arse if there is blood in the butt or cuts in the mouth.

- Sucking dick without a condom when there are mouth wounds, bleeding gums, throat infections, or cuts on the cock.

- Fingering and fisting the arse causing damage to the inside lining, or when fingers, hands or arms have cuts or abrasions.

- Sharing enemas, flogging implements or sex toys that go inside the body, break the skin or which have cum, blood or serum on them.

- Pissing in the eyes, ears, nose, mouth or arse, or on open wounds or skin rashes.

- Shitting in the mouth, or on broken skin.

Unsafest sex

- Fucking arse without a condom.

Sexy Without Risk
HIV Safer sex checklist

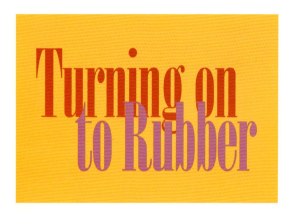

Cum in a condom

Condoms can be sexy. It depends on your attitude. If you think positive and see rubbers as an erotic sex toy which can save you a lot of worry, and also save your life, then you'll find using them a positive experience. If you have HIV, condoms enable you to have raunchy sex secure in the knowledge that you're not putting your partner at risk.

Men who have difficulty getting used to wearing condoms should experiment with different brands and styles. Some are more comfortable than others. With practice, using condoms is as natural as using lube. They become an integral part of sex.

Many guys get so used to sticking on a rubber that they develop an erotic association between rubbers and orgasms. The mere sight of a condom produces added stiffness and excitement. Rubbers become a turn-on in their own right. They signal that the build-up to orgasm is about to begin – and that signal is very arousing.

There are plenty of guys who get a special sexual kick out of the tightness of condoms. They find the pressure on their prick incredibly sexy. Others turn on to the smell and taste of condoms. These rubber fetishists just love the unique latex sensations of condomized sex. Some guys get a big thrill from having their partner put a condom on them. The feel of another man rolling a rubber down their cock shaft, with his hands or his lips, drives them wild.

Anxiety about HIV is a big passion-killer. Using a condom gives us protection and security. This means we can focus our minds on sexual bliss. A lot of guys cum too quick. By reducing sensitivity slightly, condoms prolong staying power and pleasure. The result is a delayed, but often much more intense, orgasm.

Be prepared

Life is full of surprises! There is always a special excitement about a chance meeting with a fabulous dreamy guy on a train or bus, in a park or museum, at a business meeting or football match. Sometimes these unforeseen encounters end up with passionate embraces in a park, toilet or alleyway. When you are both frantic to fuck, it is very frustrating to have to say no because you left your condoms at home. So don't forget: be prepared for that unexpected adventure. Carry condoms and lube wherever you go. Always keep some in your wallet, jacket, jeans, briefcase, sports bag and car. You never know when you may need them.

Carrying rubbers doesn't mean you are easy or sleazy. It means you are sexy and smart, that you care about yourself and others, and that you are ready to take full advantage of a sudden opportunity for some great safe fucking.

At home, keep condoms and lube everywhere. There's nothing more infuriating than not being able to find them when you need them. Stash some by the bed and sofa, and in the fridge and bathroom cabinet. That way, whenever lust overwhelms you, condoms and lube will be close to hand.

Which is safest?

When used correctly, condoms offer almost 100% protection against HIV – and many other infections. However, not all rubbers are of perfect quality. Some can have faults which can lead to breakage.

Rubber tips

For the most reliable condoms:

✇ Choose a well-known brand. These tend to be better made, and more rigorously tested for faults.

✇ Stick to condoms that are marked 'electronically tested' and which carry a quality control kitemark and an expiry date.

✇ Use only 'ultra-strong' or 'extra strong' rubbers when you screw. The lighter-weight versions are not suitable for arse-fucking and tear more easily. Flavoured condoms are for sucking only, and are not tough enough for screwing.

✇ Buy from reputable stores or supermarkets. Because they trade on their public image, these stores are more likely to sell rubbers which meet stringent safety standards and have been tested properly.

✇ Get your condoms from busy highstreet stores or supermarkets. The rapid turnover of stock means their condoms are newer; they are less likely to have been sitting on the shelf for ages.

✇ Avoid animal skin condoms. They are not as tough as rubber, and they are not as effective in stopping the transfer of HIV and other infections.

✇ Be wary of novelty condoms and unknown brands. Their quality is sometimes inferior to that of standard rubbers and nationally-known brand names.

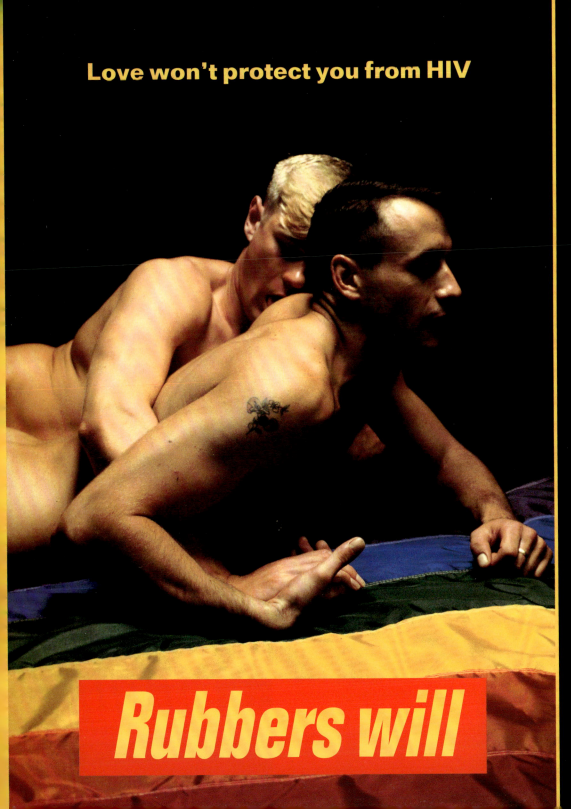

Love won't protect you from HIV

Rubbers will

Turning on to Rubber
Lubrication

Varieties and styles

Condoms come in many shapes, colours, textures and flavours – just like dicks. Strong and elastic, they will stretch to cover any size cock, no matter how huge. A strong rubber has an expansion capacity sufficient to hold 20 litres of water!

Standard condoms are uncoloured and transparent. However, you can also get them in virtually every colour of the rainbow. They come in various shapes: straight-sided, flared and bulbous. You can find tentacled and ribbed versions to give extra sensation to the person being screwed, although these are rarely of the 'extra strong' variety and therefore unsuitable for arse-screwing.

Many condoms have a small teat at the end to collect the spunk after you cum. Others have a plain rounded end that gives a snugger fit. There are rubbers with lubrication to smooth penetration when fucking, and some have spermicide to kill HIV. For sucking dick, unlubricated condoms without spermicide taste better. Or, try a flavoured condom.

Lubrication

Your arse does not have sufficient natural moisture to ensure a juicy, safe fuck. Even lubricated condoms are not wet and slippery enough. Added lube is necessary to ease penetration and thrusting, and to protect the rubber against damage.

Lack of adequate lube causes dryness and friction, which is uncomfortable. Friction can damage your arse and can cause the condom to split.

Avoid using oil-based lubricants such as vaseline, butter, margarine, crisco, moisturizing cream, petroleum jelly, baby oil and hand lotion. The oil in these lubes rapidly weakens condoms and causes them to disintegrate or split. Always read the label on your lube to make sure it contains no oil. Choose a

Safer Sexy
Turning on to Rubber

water-based lube, such as KY jelly, which is oil-free.

When the condom is on your dick, add lots of lube to the rubber, and also to the outside and inside of your partner's arse-hole to get him wet and fuckable. During prolonged sex, lube can dry out. So you may need to add an extra dab to keep yourselves moist.

Spit (saliva) isn't a good lube for fucking. It isn't smooth and silky enough. Using spit can cause friction, which doesn't feel good and may cause a condom to burst. There is also a small danger that spit might contain traces of blood infected with HIV or other diseases (if you have mouth wounds).

Some guys like to use lubrication when jerking off together. Those who have been circumcised may need some lube to get themselves going. Others just prefer the different sensation that lube gives. If you use lubrication when jerking off, avoid using your partner's cum on your own dick. It might get inside your dick-hole and expose you to the risk of infection.

It is safest to lube yourself from squeeze tubes or squirt-top dispensers. These types of containers prevent your lube supply from becoming contaminated. Lube in jars could, in theory, spread infection if partners dip their fingers into the jar after having been up an arse or after having got cum on their hands while jerking off. But this risk is, of course, a tiny one.

Spermicides

Spermicides are chemicals that kill sperm. Many condoms are now coated with spermicides containing Nonoxynol-9, which can destroy HIV and other infections. Some lubricants also include a spermicide that can kill HIV. This is, however, much less effective than a condom in preventing HIV.

Spermicides offer extra protection in case a rubber breaks. So always use a spermicide *together* with a condom. Never use a spermicide *instead* of a condom.

Some guys are allergic to spermicides. They get red, sore and itchy in the arse or on the dick. Apart from the discomfort, these signs can mean the skin is damaged. This can make it easier for HIV to penetrate the affected area if the condom slips off or tears open. If you have a bad reaction to a spermicide, stop using it immediately.

You can test whether you are allergic to a spermicide by unrolling a condom and rubbing it on your cock or arse. Check hourly over a few hours. If you notice any inflammation or irritation, switch to a condom with a different spermicide, or try a brand that is spermicide-free.

Protecting condoms

♂ Store your condoms in a dry, cool and dark place. They can be damaged by heat, damp and ultra-violet light. This means you need to keep rubbers away from radiators, lamps and direct sunshine.

♂ It is also best not to leave condoms for long periods in warm places, such as the glove compartment of a car or on top of a television or music system.

♂ Carry rubbers with you wherever you go, but avoid keeping them for weeks in your pocket or wallet where they can get damaged by coins or keys.

Always check the expiry date on the packet – never use condoms that are out of date.

Condom sense

Fucking a guy in the arse is a great way to cum. Being fucked is also a fabulous sensation. Using a condom ensures fucking euphoria, with security. Screwing

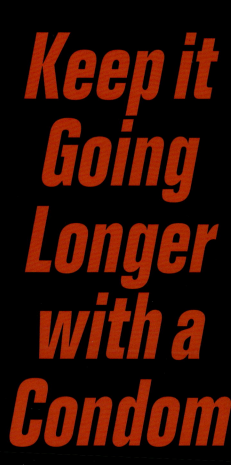

Condoms prolong staying power

Keep it Going Longer with a Condom

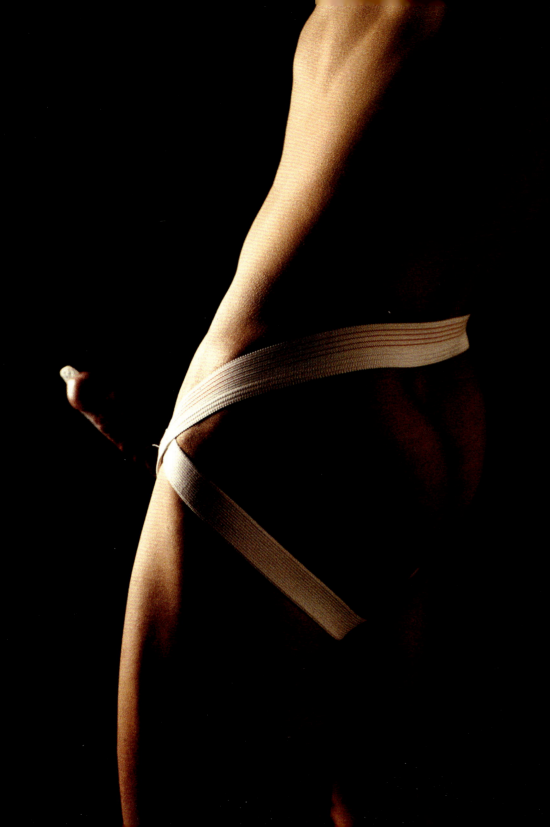

Turning on to Rubber
Putting it on and taking it off

safely with a condom is more important than all the other safer sex acts put together. It will radically reduce your likelihood of getting or passing on HIV. If everyone fucked with a rubber, the AIDS epidemic would be dramatically arrested. Thousands of gay lives could be saved, perhaps including your own and those of your friends and lovers. You can strike a blow against HIV by fucking safe forever.

If you intend to screw, put on a condom as soon as you get hard. This doesn't mean you have to cum immediately. It is just a lot easier to pause at the beginning of sex to roll on a rubber than later in the middle of frenzied passion. Putting on a condom from the moment you are hard also protects against pre-cum, which can contain HIV. For cock-sucking, it is wise to use a condom if there are cuts or sores in the mouth, or on the dick.

Putting it on and taking it off

Using a condom correctly ensures that you stay fucking safe.

⚣ Your dick deserves the best. Choose a strong and reputable brand of condom which is marked 'electronically tested' or has a logo showing that it meets approved standards of reliability.

⚣ Check the date on the condom wrapping to make sure it hasn't expired.

⚣ Open the packet carefully with your hands, not with your teeth or scissors. Take care not to damage the rubber with nails, rings or bits of rough skin.

⚣ Be sure your cock is dry and free of lubrication before you put the condom on, otherwise it may slip off when you fuck.

Safer Sexy
Turning on to Rubber

- Check that you are holding the rubber the right way round.

- Squeeze the teat at the closed end of the condom between your thumb and forefinger to expel any air. If your condom hasn't got a teat, squeeze the top centimetre to make a reservoir for your cum.

- If you are uncircumsized, pull back your foreskin. By now you should be swollen and stiff in anticipation of the fuck to come. If you are not, get your partner to lick your balls and play with your prick to make you horny.

- When you are rock hard, put the condom on the head of your cock to cover your piss-hole.

- Roll the rubber all the way down the shaft of your dick to the base, or better still get your partner to do it for you. If you use your lips and tongue to roll a condom on another guy's cock, make sure you don't damage it with your teeth.

- Stroke the shaft with firm downward movements to smooth out any wrinkles in the condom, and to keep your dick hard and excited.

- Add plenty of water-based lubricant, such as KY, to your condom-covered dick to get it slippery and ready for fucking. Don't use oil.

- Guide your cock into your partner's arse-hole, penetrating very slowly and gently at first, then gradually plunging harder, faster and deeper as you feel his arse muscles relax around your shaft.

- During long sex sessions, check regularly that the condom is still on and has not ripped. Add extra lube if you start feeling dry.

- When all the safety aspects are taken care of, you can get on with the business of pumping, gasping, kissing, sweating and thrusting to orgasmic ecstasy.

- Soon after cumming, and while you are still hard, slowly pull your prick out of his arse. Hold the condom tight at the base of your cock to stop it slipping off or any cum leaking out.

- Tie a knot in the used condom, wrap it in tissue paper, and put it in a rubbish bin (not down the toilet, as this causes blockages). Then relax in his arms. Paradise!

Remember

- Be careful to avoid oil-based lubricants such as vaseline and moisterizing cream, which weaken rubbers and cause them to disintegrate. Always use a water-based lube, like KY jelly.

- If you don't like the dry constricted feeling of condoms, try adding three pea-sized drops of lubricant inside the tip of the rubber. This creates a moist, slippery feeling which can enhance the sensitivity of the top of the dick during screwing. Use just enough to make the head of your cock wet inside the condom. Don't add too much lube or let it get down the shaft of your dick – as this could cause the condom to slip off.

- If you accidentally put a rubber on the wrong way round, and find it will not roll down the shaft, never turn it up the right way and use it. This could leave infectious fluid from your dick-hole on the outside of the condom, which might put your partner at risk. To be safe, throw the condom away and use a new one.

- Warts on the dick or arse can sometimes damage condoms. Get them treated.

- It is not safe to re-use condoms. They're not strong enough and re-use can spread infection. When you fuck again, always put on a new condom.

- Condoms very rarely tear if you use them correctly. But if this possibility worries you, *in addition to wearing a condom*, try withdrawing your dick before you cum.

Latex barriers

Licking, kissing or tonguing a guy's arse-hole can be incredibly erotic and a deliriously pleasurable way of exciting a man as a prelude to fucking him. However, it can also involve a risk of getting Hepatitis A and B, gonorrhoea, intestinal parasites such as amoebiasis, and possibly HIV if there is blood in or around his butt-hole. Latex barriers, also known as dental dams, can help protect you against these risks when you eat out another guy's arse.

Made out of ultra-fine rubber, similar to condoms, latex barriers are about 15 centimetres or 6 inches square. Held against your partner's arse while your tongue slides over and into his hole, they form a protective shield between him and your mouth. This reduces the risk of transmitting disease from his arse to your mouth, and vice versa.

If you don't like the taste of rubber, try using a fruit-flavoured latex barrier, or add your own flavouring using honey, yoghurt, or chocolate. To enhance the sensations for the guy you are tonguing in the arse, add a little water-based lubrication to his arse-hole before you put the latex barrier against it.

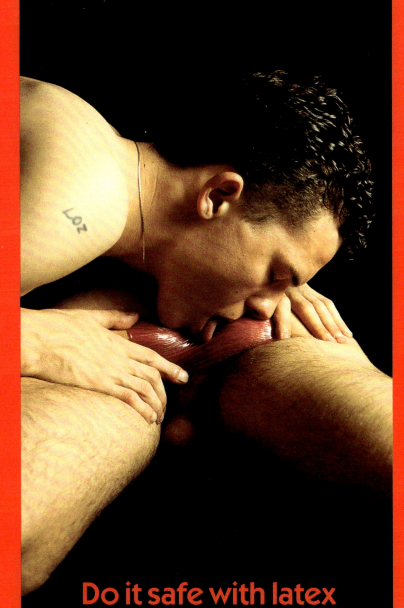

Smart Arse Lickers

Do it safe with latex

Turning on to Rubber
Latex barriers

If you haven't got a latex barrier, you can make one:

🔖 Choose a fruit-flavoured condom, or a plain condom if you prefer funky arse-hole aromas.

🔖 Unroll the condom.

🔖 With a pair of scissors, cut it lengthways down one side.

🔖 Spread the cut condom flat on your partner's arse, and get licking!

🔖 If you prefer, wash off any lubrication and spermicide with cold soapy water before you apply the condom to his arse.

In an emergency, when there is nothing else available, you can use kitchen cling-film. But you need to be careful because it's not very strong and tends to break with vigorous tonguing.

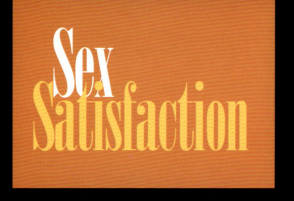

Sex Satisfaction

Truly sensational sex happens only occasionally. Sustained sensational sex, time after time, is much harder to achieve – particularly when you have been together with the same partner for a long time. In permanent relationships, it is all too easy for sex to become routine and matter of fact.

There is no magic formula for sensual success, either with a new partner or a long-established one. However, there are things you can do to increase the chances of a good quality sex life.

Communicating desires

Erotic fulfilment depends on sending the right signals to the guy you are with, and understanding the signals he is sending to you. Let your partner know your likes and dislikes. Show your approval and encouragement when he does something that turns you on. Gasp and writhe with pleasure. Smile. Kiss him. Ask for more. Otherwise, he will never know what you like.

Don't put up with things you don't enjoy. If you hate sucking with a condom, suggest an alternative. Or, manoeuvre your body into a new position and start doing something else.

Observation and imitation

Watch your fuckmate's eyes, facial expressions and body language. Listen to his breathing. His reactions can tell you whether he is getting off on what you are doing, or merely putting up with it. Note what he does to you. Usually, it signifies what he likes having done to him. If he licks your arse, respond in kind. Imitation and mutuality also evoke feelings of intimacy and empathy. Many guys find this gives added enjoyment to a sexual encounter, no matter how fleeting.

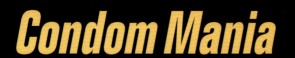

Condom Mania — Riskless Rapture

Refuse to use condoms?

Sex Satisfaction — **Danger-free**

Sameness or difference?

Good sex doesn't need identical erotic interests. Nor does it need diametrically opposed attractions. Both sexual sameness and sexual difference can be compatible. Each can form the basis for sizzling passion. If you both like the same type of sex, it is a great boon. A shared fixation for a particular activity like being fucked, or bondage, is not a problem providing both of you are versatile and don't mind taking it in turns.

Two completely opposite guys can also gel together, the one complementing the other. When a man who loves to suck cock has a relationship with a man who loves to be sucked, their different tastes produce mutual hard-on happiness.

Reciprocation

Give and take is necessary for the success of any liaison, including the briefest and the longest. Shared enjoyment makes for the best sex. It is impossible to sustain one-sided satisfaction indefinitely. If one person is not fulfiled, it sooner or later dulls the excitement for both and dampens the action all round. Conversely, when two guys sexually bewitch each other, it escalates the erotic intensity for both of them. Make sure you give your partner plenty of stimulation; getting him all fired up will encourage him to fire you up too.

Diversity

Sticking to a narrow range of sexual acts may make it hard to find a man you click with. With a limited menu, sex can become boring – if not for you, then perhaps for your partner. It also means that you miss out on a lot of arousing sensations, some of which you may really enjoy if you bother to try them. A large and diverse sensual repertoire helps keep sex feeling fresh and thrilling. It also broadens your options for libidinous pleasure, and increases your chances of compatibility with a new partner.

Inventiveness

Being creative between the sheets can do a lot to invigorate a relationship. In contrast, a lack of sexual imagination can be very tedious and a sure-fire route to divorce.

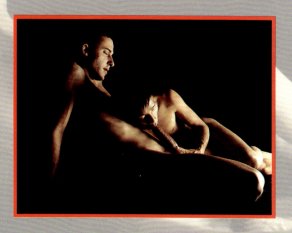

Try new ways of doing favourite activities. Fuck him in an arm chair or in a sling for a change. Incorporate novelties like toys and food into your humping and pumping. Experiment with forms of sex you have never tried before, such as bondage and thigh rubbing.

Avoidance of routine

Predictability deadens the loins. While everyone can enjoy a tried and trusted sexual routine for a time, eventually it loses its shine. Spontaneity and adventure can, however, prolong the momentum of a passionate affair.

Initiate sex when and where your partner least expects it. In the shower first thing in the morning. Behind the tool shed when he's in the middle of gardening. In the back seat of the car on the way to visit your parents. Over the kitchen sink while he's peeling the carrots. Anything to escape from an everyday humdrum sexual routine.

Versatility

Guys who confine themselves to one particular sex role deny themselves a bunch of fun. Lack of adaptability can drive boyfriends rigid – with boredom, not arousal. If being spanked and screwed is the limit of your erotic appetite, that's fine providing it satisfies both you and your partner. Flexibility, however, has its rewards. A willingness to swing both ways gives you the best of both worlds: active and passive, top and bottom. This can mean new sexual kicks, some of which you might enjoy.

Danger-free

Avoiding risky sex acts, especially fucking without a condom, gives both him and you protection. It ensures peace of mind. On the other hand, unsafe behaviour often leads to post-sex anxiety about HIV. It ruins the after-glow and corrodes a relationship.

Worrying if your man has the virus and if he has given it to you fosters suspicion and undermines trust. It's so unnecessary. Safer sex banishes the need for worry, distrust and suspicion. It doesn't matter if either of you has HIV. Steering clear of dangerous acts gives you both the confidence and security to concentrate on achieving sexual nirvana.

Suck! don't Fuck!

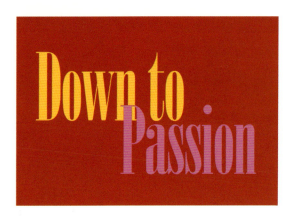

Down to Passion

Long before we get around to cumming, there are lots of preliminary sexual activities which can give us great satisfaction: kissing, fingering, massaging, licking, caressing and much more. Sometimes disparaged as 'foreplay', these activities are pleasures in their own right and they help stoke the fires of erotic heat. Sex without them is much less interesting and passionate. What's more, they are either totally safe or very low-risk.

Erogenous zones

Flesh is synonymous with sensuality. The entire surface of our body is teeming with billions of sensual nerve-endings. All have incredible erotic potential – when stimulated in the right way. These diverse sites of carnal pleasure, known as 'erogenous' zones, crave stimulation and contribute to the process of sexual arousal and orgasmic explosion. Good sex is about more than the enjoyment we get from our dicks and arses. It is a whole-body experience in which the stimulation of many different erogenous zones combine to produce climactic ecstasy.

The sensitivity of different erogenous zones varies from person to person. It is a matter of exploring your body to discover which parts turn you on the strongest. Some of the main erogenous zones are: the lips, nose, eye-lids, forehead, ear, back and base of the neck, spine, shoulders, arm-pits, inside of the arm, wrists, palms, fingertips, nipples, sides of the chest below the arm-pits, stomach, navel, groin, testicles, buttocks, sphincter, inside of the thigh, back of the knee, ankles, soles of the feet, and toe tips.

The means of stimulating these erogenous zones are as varied as your imagination: use your hands, lips, tongue, breath, hair and feet. Try a feather, ice-cube or fern frond. Caress with clothes made of lace, rubber, fake fur, silk, leather or mohair. Discover the delights of hair dryers and vibrators.

Kissing

If dicks are about lust, lips involve feelings. Kissing combines sex with emotion. It is an expression of intimacy and affection, as well as raw desire. When a guy kisses a lot, it's usually a sign of an emotional charge as well as a sexual one. Conversely, an absence or infrequency of kissing normally signifies emotional detachment, ambivalence about a relationship, or hang-ups about being gay.

A really good kiss is dripping wet, using both the lips and tongue to explore a guy's whole mouth. Try this: caress his tongue with yours. Massage the gums under his upper and lower lips. Tickle the roof of his

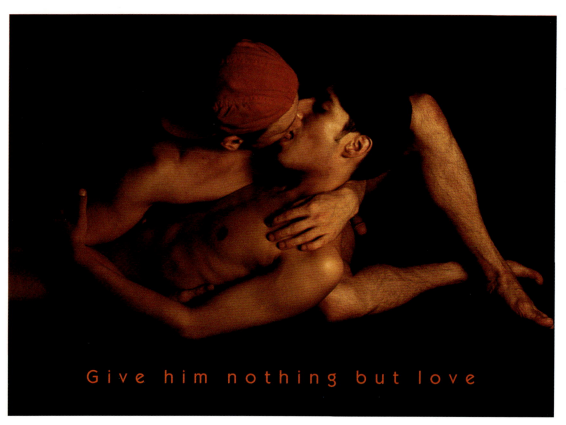

Give him nothing but love

mouth. Fondle the fleshy area under his tongue. Nibble his lips. For extra thrills, fill your mouth with beer or champagne and, as you kiss, slowly dribble it into your partner's mouth. Or pass a chocolate back and forth, from mouth to mouth, while you are kissing.

There are, of course, many places to kiss a guy other than on his mouth. Every inch of his body, from head to toe, is kissable. Passionate all-over wet kisses will have him writhing and groaning with delight.

Safe kissing

The risk of HIV from kissing is negligible. Although spit can contain the virus, the amounts are too small to be infectious. It would take exposure to two or three litres of spit to put a person at risk of HIV. Spit also contains substances which help neutralize and inactivate HIV. Not surprisingly, nobody anywhere in the world has ever been shown to have got HIV from kissing. The only conceivable risk, and it is a very long-shot, is that HIV could be transmitted between guys who kiss when they both have open cuts and bleeding in their mouths. This is, however, exceedingly unlikely. Indeed, there has not been a single recorded case of it ever happening. For all intents and purposes, kissing is no risk for HIV.

Nevertheless, if you feel the need to be ultra safe, avoid wet kissing if you and your partner both have open cuts or bleeding in your mouths or on your lips.

Food

Food gives added flavour to your sex life. It makes kissing and licking another guy's body a truly delicious experience. All you have to do is choose a food you really enjoy and spread it liberally on the body parts you want to kiss and lick. The possibili-

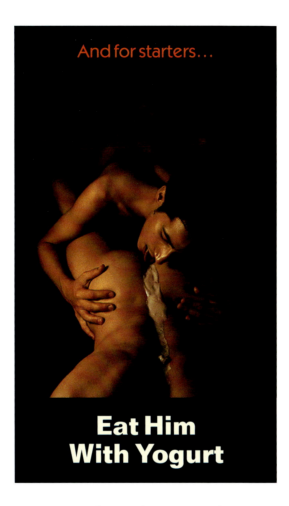

And for starters…

Eat Him With Yogurt

ties are as endless as the contents of your cupboards and refrigerator: raspberry jam, whipped cream, wild honey, banana yogurt, maple syrup, pineapple ice cream or melted chocolate. If you use oily foods, keep them away from condoms as oil damages rubber.

Dip his cock and balls in blackcurrant juice. Smother his toes with double cream. Fill his armpits with lemon sorbet. Cover his arse-hole with peanut butter. Then get licking!

Love-bites

When he wants sensations a little harder than your lips and tongue can offer, try using your teeth. Gently nibble his ears or balls. Nip him around the arse and ankles. Try a slow, firm chew of his tits or toes. If he enjoys that, give him some love-bites on the neck and nipples. Start gently and ever so gradually increase the pressure of your bite. Note his reaction. Unless you know he enjoys pain, don't bite so hard that it hurts him. A good love-bite should be a delectable pleasure tinged with very mild pain. Avoid love-bites which break the skin – as blood can transmit HIV.

Caressing

Touching and caressing are key physical stimulants which trigger sexual arousal. Feeling the body of a guy you fancy, and being felt by him, produces a surge of erotic hormones and a rush of blood to your loins. With caressing, it can sometimes be the case that less means more. While firm and frenzied caresses can be arousing, softness and lightness of touch can also be very sensual. Barely touching the skin, just skimming the hairs on the surface, sends many of us into exhilarating rapture.

Like kissing, caressing is expressive of emotional feelings, not just sexual sensations. A lack or brevity of touch suggests indifference about a person. Rough handling, unless it is part of a mutually agreed sado-masochistic scene, may denote feelings of anger, resentment and contempt. In contrast, frequent soft caresses and warm embraces are very calming and relaxing. They also indicate feelings of closeness and tenderness. Many guys find this gives an added passionate intensity to sex. Affectionate touches can make the sexual act more than a mere physical release, even during a one-night stand.

Down to Passion — Safer Sexy

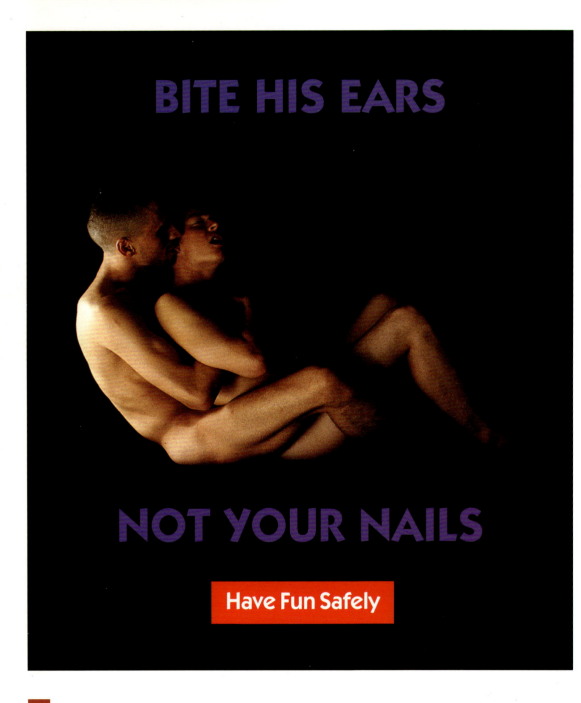

Massage

Massage is a fun and effective way to ease body aches and pains, and it relieves stress and anxiety. It can also be an erotically-charged preliminary to sex, stirring carnal desires and stimulating sexual appetite. Try the following:

✧ Rub your hands together vigorously to generate heat, then apply oil – massage oil, baby oil, bath oil, olive oil – to your partner's body.

✧ As you massage, alternate between using different parts of your hands: your open palm and knuckles, and your finger and thumb tips.

✧ Vary your massage technique from kneading the flesh to rapid chopping movements, circular motions, and rhythmic on-off pressure.

✧ For maximum erotic effect, concentrate on the back of the neck, ears, nipples, waist, groin, buttocks, inside of arms and thighs, fingers, ankles, toes, and soles of the feet.

✧ As well as using your hands, try massaging with a smooth billiard ball, rolling pin, or large coke bottle filled with hot (or cold) water.

✧ Experiment with different oils and lotions. Peppermint gives an all-over tingly sensation. Keep massage oils away from his arse and your cock if you intend to fuck (oil rots rubbers).

Fingering

Fingering a man's arse is often a prelude to screwing him, as it helps relax and open his butt-hole. But it's also bliss in itself. A good fingering excites the prostate gland, and makes a sensual, and safe, substitute for fucking.

Begin by moistening his arse-hole and your finger

Down to Passion
Fingering

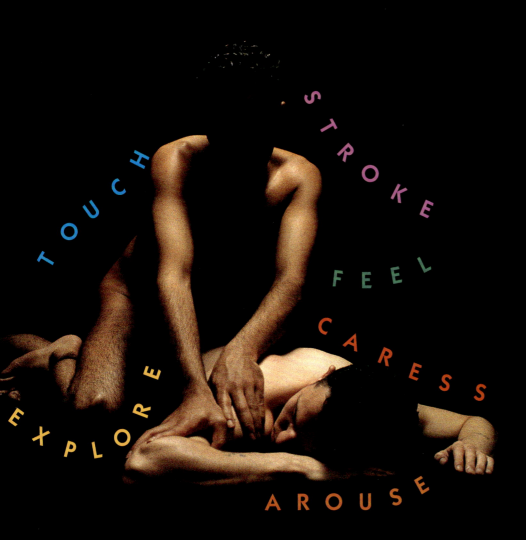

TOUCH STROKE FEEL CARESS AROUSE EXPLORE

with some lube. Softly tease and tickle his opening with your finger-tips. Poke your finger against his hole, using gentle on-off pressure. Gradually quicken the tempo of your probing. As you feel his muscles loosening, bit-by-bit penetrate your finger inside him. Enjoy the sensation of his hot, wet flesh closing around your finger. When you sense he is fully relaxed, finger-fuck him using slow, long, deep thrusting movements. Or, try twisting corkscrew motions. Pause every now and then to stroke the inner lining of his arse and to massage his sexually-excitable prostate gland, which lies behind the pubic bone. If he likes a bigger feeling, add extra fingers. Unlike fucking, fingering is something you can both do to each other at the same time. You can also do it while simultaneously sucking dick, rubbing bodies and jerking off together.

Safe fingering

Fingering is normally no risk for HIV. The only possible ways the virus could be transferred are if you have open cuts on your finger, or if you swop your finger between his arse and your arse (and vice versa). If you are anxious:

- Use a different finger or rubber gloves, when you have a cut.

- Only finger one arse, yours or his, but not both.

- Keep your fingernails short and smooth to prevent damage to the delicate membranes of the arse.

- Remove any rings prior to finger insertion.

- When you get cum or pre-cum on your hands, always wash them thoroughly before you stick them up anyone's arse.

- If you have warts on your fingers or hands, don't put them inside your partner's butt – as you might give him the wart virus. Get warts treated pronto.

Safer Sexy
Down to Passion

Licking arse

Licking arse is known as 'rimming' in gay slang, and as 'anilingus' in medical jargon. It is one of the most sensual of all gay sex acts. The skin around the arsehole is gloriously sensitive. Having it kissed or tongued, makes most men squeal with exhilaration.

Start by getting your partner to lie face down on his stomach. Run your tongue up and down his spine, from his neck to his butt-hole. Blow gently on the wet trail you have left behind. Then kiss and massage his buttocks. Tickle his crack with your fingers. Softly tug the hairs around his hole. Give him a few light bites on the arse. Dribble some spit in between his cheeks. Wriggle your tongue into the crack. Nibble the muscles around his opening. Get off on the sensation of them relaxing and contracting. Move your tongue in ever-smaller spirals around his arse-hole. When you reach the opening, push your tongue inside. Thrust deeper and deeper with each penetration. Lick him inside. Feel his butt twitching with erotic delirium. A variant position for rimming is having a guy sit on your face. This allows maximum tongue penetration, together with an element of domination and humiliation, if that's your bag. Another option is the pleasure of mutual rimming where two guys in the '69' position simultaneously eat each other's arses.

Rimming, like fingering, helps relax the arse muscles and eroticizes the arse-hole, leaving many men craving to be screwed senseless. This makes it a very good warm-up activity if you want to fuck.

Arse-Hole Ecstasy

Low-Risk for HIV

Safe arse-licking

Slurping arse is very low-risk for HIV, even if you poke your tongue right up a guy's butt-hole. However, it is high-risk for hepatitis and intestinal diseases such as amoebiasis. Be arse smart: get vaccinated against hepatitis A and B.

With regard to HIV, it's up to you to consider the very small risk involved in rimming and decide whether it is a risk you're willing to take. It's extremely unlikely that arse juices could pass on HIV, unless they contain infected blood. Only a handful of men in the entire world are suspected to have got the virus from rimming. Nevertheless, if you want to opt for no-risk rather than low-risk, and protect yourself against other arse-borne diseases:

- Shower before rimming and only lick the outside of the arse-hole.

- Fingering and fucking leave germs on the outside of the arse. It's therefore safest to rim *before* you finger or fuck, rather than afterwards.

- Use a latex barrier when you penetrate your tongue inside his butt, if you have cuts in your mouth, or if your partner has arse fissures or bleeding piles (haemorrhoids).

Tit play

Nipples can be a source of great sexual pleasure and excitation, sometimes becoming firm and erect. Tit play involves tweaking the nipples to get them sensualized and aroused. There are lots of different techniques you can use:

- Caressing, pulling, rubbing and pinching.

- Licking and blowing on the moistened skin.

- Kissing, sucking, nibbling and biting.

If you are more adventurous, massage the nipples with a vibrator or electric toothbrush. Stroke them with an ice-cube or a hot spoon. Or squeeze them with tit clamps (which you can always improvise with clothes-pegs for example).

Noise

When the guy you are sexing does something you really enjoy, let him know. Gasp and moan with delight. Whisper exclamations of approval and encouragement: 'Yes!' 'Great!' 'More!' Call out your partner's name or scream that you love him. Talk romantic or shout dirty: 'Fuck me! Harder! Faster!'

Whatever way you do it, communicate your pleasure. This enables your partner to figure out what sort of stimulation drives you wildest. If he knows what you like, he can concentrate on giving you more of it. If you don't tell him, he may move on to another activity which might be less fun.

Noisy sex can be a terrific turn-on. Many of us get off on the lewd squelching, slurping sounds of fucking and sucking. We also find that squeals of passionate frenzy from our fuckmate ignites sexual fever in us. This sets in motion a reciprocal response. One partner gets excited and he gasps and moans, whispers and yells. These noises make his partner excited. He too responds with excited noises. Each partner's cries of passion spurs the other to new heights of sexual ecstasy.

Make plenty of noise during sex. Breathing deeply and heavily, and groaning with joy, helps to relax your whole body and release inhibitions. Try it. Breathe deeply. As you exhale, let out moans of pleasure. When you cum, scream with lascivious delight. Vocalizing your lust and emotions in this way can result in intensified sexual sensations and stronger orgasms.

Sex toys

Sex toys do what you want, when you want. They never complain, have a headache, or stand you up. Whether you use them as a substitute for a regular partner, to spice up a jaded relationship, or just for the sheer enjoyment of something different and exciting, sex toys can be a very obliging and fun addition to your erotic inventory. Try experimenting with cock rings, whips, dildoes, tit clamps, butt plugs, handcuffs, vibrators, canes, and ball constrainers. Or improvise your own with paper clamps, leather straps, and phallic-shaped fruit and vegetables.

You'll find that sex toys can often help increase sexual excitement and enable the exploration of new sexual possibilities. Cock rings make a semi-stiff dick rock hard, prolong erections, and create a unique tight feeling around the prick and balls. A dildo simulates the fullness of having a cock up your arse while allowing you to suck off your partner at the same time. Tit clamps produce a sharper pain than squeezing the nipples with your fingers, and they leave your hands free to pursue other desires.

Dildoes are the most popular gay sex toy. They give you the enjoyment of being screwed, without the worry of HIV. They also allow you to choose the size and shape of what is going inside you, and to control the pace and depth of the penetration. If you want to make your own dildo, choose a vegetable like a cucumber (or a corn cob if you prefer ticklish ribbed sensations). Use a knife to round off the end and remove any rough bits. Soaking it in warm water for a couple of minutes helps create a steamy dick sensation when you slip it in. But do not use hot water or leave it soaking for too long as this could cause it to break half way through the action. Before you push your vegetable dildo in, lubricate it well. If you get an adverse reaction from the vegetable skin, or if you plan to use it afterwards for dinner, cover it completely with a condom before you thrust it inside.

Safe sex toys

Have fun with toys but keep it risk free:

🌈 Because the lining of the arse is easily damaged, objects inserted into the butt-hole often pick up traces of blood or mucus which may be infected with HIV or other sexually-transmitted diseases.

🌈 Always clean sex toys after use, as dirty ones spread germs.

🌈 Sex toys that go up the arse, break the skin, or get blood, serum or cum on them, should not be shared with other guys. Get your own set and keep toys to yourself. When you visit a lover, take your toys with you.

🌈 If you do use someone else's sex toys, wash them in hot soapy water, soak them in strong disinfectant for at least 30 minutes, and then rinse them thoroughly under running water. Alternatively, if you are swapping arse toys, put a new condom on them every time they get passed from one guy to another.

🌈 Choose dildoes, butt plugs and vibrators that are made of smooth, pliable and soft rubber or plastic to prevent damage to your arse. Avoid inserting objects that are sharp, breakable, pointy, rough, hard or inflexible.

🌈 Make sure that whatever you put inside your arse is no longer than 25 centimetres or 10 inches (the most an arse can safely take), and that it has a wide base or rope to stop it disappearing inside you – otherwise you might well end up in hospital getting it surgically removed.

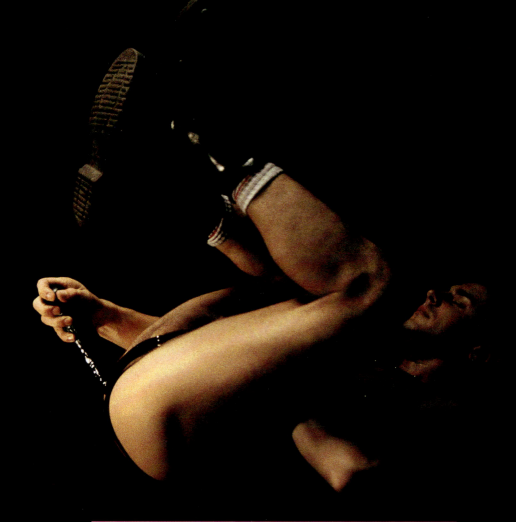

Toys Are Sexy

And they don't throw tantrums or leave you for another guy!

Down to Passion
Fantasy

Fantasy

Sexual fantasies have three great attractions. They are totally self-controlled, completely private, and absolutely risk-free. You can create a fantasy to fit your exact desires: sex with the man of your dreams, in whatever location you choose, and as often as you like. The constraints of reality cease to apply. Keanu Reeves is screwable on a beach in Hawaii whenever you want. Because fantasies take place in the privacy of your own mind, no one else need know about them. You can let go of all your inhibitions and fantasize about doing things that you might never normally have the bravado to do, like having orgiastic sex in the back row of a crowded cinema.

Fantasies also have the advantage that once they are over it's instant goodbye! You don't have to go through any polite rituals to get rid of a guy you'd rather not see again, and you never suffer the disappointment of a fabulous fuck not phoning like he said he would!

A fantasy is nothing more than a mental image. This means it's a very safe form of sex. There is no danger of HIV if we day-dream about swallowing the cum of the hunky pizza delivery boy or sucking out the arse-juices of the cute plumber's mate. However, as well as the fantasies that stay in our heads, there are also the fantasies we act out with a partner. These may, for example, involve dressing up in uniforms and simulating fucking a hot motorcycle cop. If acted-out fantasies include unsafe acts, there can be a risk of HIV. Occasional fantasies about violent or unsafe sex are usually harmless. Most guys can distinguish very clearly between fantasy and reality. They don't get confused, and don't overstep the limits of consensual role-playing. Sometimes fantasies can even provide a safety valve for sexual frustrations. But when fantasies of rape and unprotected sex become obsessive, and tempt guys to act them out for real, then they become very dangerous. Anyone

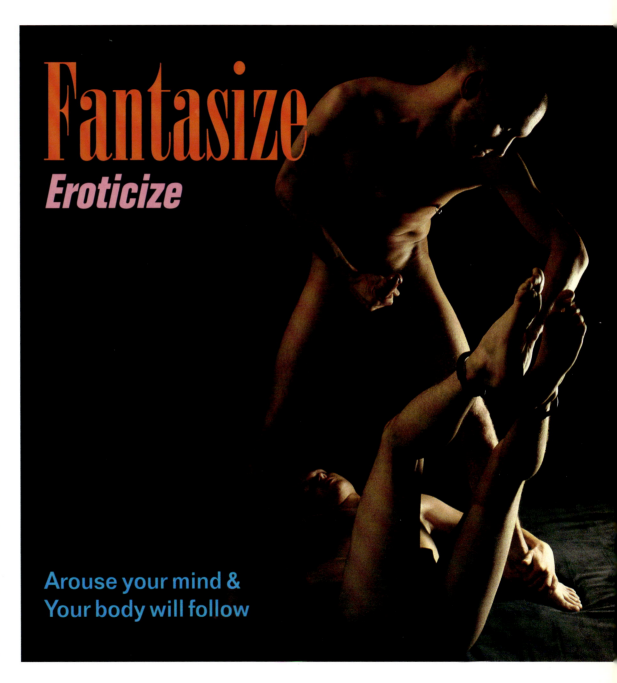

Fantasize
Eroticize

**Arouse your mind &
Your body will follow**

Safer Sexy
Down to Passion

in that situation should seek professional counselling immediately.

Most fantasies revolve around two basic scenarios. First, reliving a particularly memorable sexual experience, like being sucked off in the school showers by the swimming captain. Second, imagining an experience we would like to have, such as being tied up and fucked by Matt Dillon or Denzel Washington. Fantasies also frequently involve acts of transgression. We may dream of doing things which are the opposite of our normal behaviour and are contrary to what is expected of us. Guys who hold positions of power and responsibility sometimes have submission and slave fantasies where they are dominated and powerless. These fantasies combine sexual release with psychological relief from the pressures of a high-powered job.

Of course, there is no single explanation for particular types of fantasies. They vary from person to person. While understanding our fantasies can give us valuable insight into ourselves, it is more important to enjoy our day-dreams and mind-games, rather than endlessly analyse them.

Exploring and expressing sexual fantasies is often a very positive experience which can:

- Enhance sexual stimulation, arousal and excitement.
- Widen and vary our erotic repertoire.
- Enliven a boring, routine sex life.
- Put us in touch with our deeper desires – and fears.
- Help heal the harmful effects of sexual repression.

Try experimenting with images of specific sexual acts (spanking, piercing, orgies), domination and humiliation (piss, torture, fisting), exotic locations (subway, mountain, prison), dangerous situations (dark alleys, toilets, train stations), celebrities (TV presenters, footballers, pop stars), rough trade (soldiers, skinheads, bikers), and guys you know (boy next door, cousin, barman).

Explore and excite

There are a huge variety of sexual acts which we can enjoy before we start on those that lead to orgasm. These acts involve minimal or no risk of HIV infection. Savour the delights of safer sex:

Begin by moistening your finger and gently running it over his lips, across his eyelids, along his nose, around the edge of his ears, down the back of his neck. Kiss him slowly, then harder. Stretch your tongue inside him to massage the roof of his mouth. Take a gulp of red wine and, pressing your lips against his, squirt it inside him. Move to his ears, licking and breathing heavily into his ear-holes. Tug at his ear-lobes with your teeth while lightly pinching his tits. Lie on top of him and kiss. Press your swollen dicks together in slow, sensuous thrusts. Feel his pre-cum wet your stomach.

Drop your head to his neck, gently biting it around the base. Then chew your way along each shoulder. Firmly run your fingers through his hair, pulling and stretching his locks as you go. Massage his scalp with small circular motions of your fingers, alternately pressing hard and soft. Trail your tongue tantalisingly around the edge of his hair-line. Then retrace the route of your tongue with gentle blows of warm, moist breath. Caress his forehead, temples and cheeks with light downward movements of your finger-tips.

Pause. Close your eyes. Fantasize about the man of your dreams. Give him a ripe-red love-bite. Sink your teeth into the side of his neck, and kiss hard. Smear some strawberry mousse over his cock and balls. Take them in your mouth. Savour the flavour. Next, roll your tongue backwards and forwards along his shoulders. Then dive down into his arm-pits. Lick and tongue them vigorously. Inhale his funky odours, while pulling his underarm hairs with your fingers. Rub an ice-cube over his nipples, down his stomach, around his groin, and along his legs.

Kiss and wet his tits, breathing heavily on the moistened area. Get your tongue turning in smaller, ever-decreasing circles around his nipples. Squeeze one nipple with your fingers, while sucking the other one with your lips. Put clothes-pegs on his tits, then flick them back and forth with your fingers. Invert your head over his body. Skim lightly across the surface of his skin with your hair. Repeat the process, using the stubble on your chin.

To get his prick steely stiff, drum your finger-tips along its length. As it bounces upwards in excitement, lick the head and catch it in your mouth. Roll him over so he is lying face down on his stomach. Wriggle your tongue up and down his spine. Blow on the wet trail left by your tongue. Take a warm, hard-boiled egg and gently caress his back; starting with his shoulders and working your way downwards over his arse, and along his legs to the soles of his feet. Then move back up to his ears. Lick them slowly all over. Chew the rear of his neck, while vigorously rubbing his scalp.

Reach down to mildly scratch him on the buttocks and thighs. Alternate between slapping and licking his butt. Give him a few sharp smacks, followed by firm manly squeezes. With a cashmere scarf or leather glove, caress his buttocks. Kiss and nibble him on the arse. Spreading the cheeks wide, smear chocolate fudge into the crack. Lick it out with big, deep slurps. Work your tongue towards his arse-hole in a spiral motion. Blow bursts of hot breath on his moistened hole. Now spread his legs wide apart and suck the area between his arse and balls. Taste the dank aromas. Turn him over again, so he is lying facing upwards on his back. Let your hand go com-

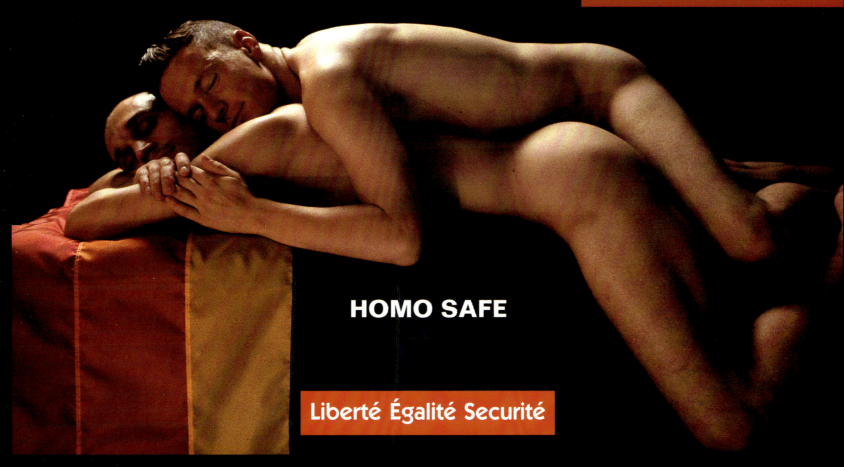

Down to Passion
Explore and excite

HOMO SAFE

Liberté Égalité Securité

pletely limp, and then use it to caress his inner forearm with barely touching backward and forward movements. Suck his fingers one by one. Lick the palm of his hand and around his wrists. Breathe softly on the wettened areas. Go down to his waist, kiss and bite him around the hips. Then trickle some spit over his engorged dick. Very slowly slide your tongue up and down the shaft. Dig your fingers hard into his shoulders. Claw the back of his head and neck, while thrusting your tongue deep inside his mouth. Next, slide your head down his chest, kissing him as you go. Stop at his groin. Poke your tongue into the tufts of pubic hair, and pull them with your lips. Move further down to his balls. One at a time, take them inside your mouth. Use your tongue to roll them around side to side, cheek to cheek.

Tickle his arse-hole with your finger, while gliding your lips over the hairs on his inner thighs. Penetrate your finger inside his arse using slow corkscrew motions. Gently stroke the wet hot flesh inside. Respond to his gasps and moans by massaging his prostate gland. Begin slowly. Then massage faster and more vigorously in synch with the increased pace of his breathing.

Lift up his legs. Nibble the back of his knee, thighs and arse. Then move your tongue along his calves to kiss his ankles and lick the soles of his feet. Press your tongue rhythmically back and forth between each toe. Then suck his toes, one by one. Be delicate at first, then suck harder. Nip the toe tips with your teeth. Lovingly blow on his wet toes as you lower his legs. Finish by warming his whole body with your hot breath; starting at his feet and working your way up to his head. Envelope his body with yours in a tender embrace.

Such fun. And so safe. Now it is his turn to do you.

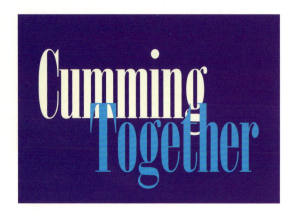

Cumming Together

Good orgasms

Getting hard and horny is triggered by many different forms of sexual stimulation:

Sight – dick, face, muscles, arse, tits.

Touch – the feel of naked flesh, caresses, massage, kissing.

Smell – fresh sweat, soap, talc, arse and cock aromas.

Taste – spit, cum, sweat.

Sound – erotic panting, pulsating music, romantic whispers, dirty talk.

Imagination – memories, wishes, fantasies.

Erotic stimuli produce arousal and excitement – an erect prick, increased blood pressure and temperature, quickened breath, dilated pupils and a surge of lust. Rubbing the cock results in escalating pleasure, the first signs of pre-cum, and faster and stronger muscle contractions. When this sexual excitement reaches peak intensity and passes beyond the point of self-control, the body is overcome with orgasm – a sudden, involuntary and immensely pleasurable release of energy which causes the dick to spurt cum. Sometimes, an orgasm is so strong that the whole body convulses with uncontrollable muscle spasms, accompanied by facial contortions and gasps of ecstatic delight. At other times, an orgasm is milder, with less body-shaking, and is confined to a strong throbbing sensation in the cock.

The quality of an orgasm depends on the pleasure experienced, and not on the method by which it is achieved. Rubbing bodies, jerking off, sucking dick and fucking arse are different ways of reaching sexual climax. None is intrinsically superior to the other. Each can produce good orgasms and bad ones. It is all down to skill and experience. This means that safer methods of sex do not have to be second rate. They can result in a climax which is just as good, or even better, than unsafe sex.

Some guys have learned how to rub bodies together in a way which produces a much more powerful orgasm than they can achieve by alternative methods. Others swear that screwing, jerking or sucking give them the best climax. The conclusion: there is no single, ultimate way to cum. With practice, one method can be just as satisfying as another.

Apart from practice, what is crucial for a good orgasm is breath and muscle control. Long and deep breaths, together with firm and rhythmic muscle contractions, help heighten and prolong the build-up to climax and the intensity of orgasmic release.

Good sex is, of course, about more than a good orgasm. It is also about good foreplay in the period before cumming. Kissing, caressing, massaging, fingering, sucking and licking are all enjoyable and fulfilling in their own right. Sometimes, they can be so satisfying that it doesn't matter if we don't cum, or if the orgasm is low-key. The crucial thing is sexual satisfaction, regardless of whether it is achieved in an orgasmic or non-orgasmic way. All that is really important is that we enjoy ourselves, safely, and feel sexually content.

Jerking off

What do you do with a dick that is engorged with blood, up-standing, rippled with veins, oozing pre-cum, and bursting to explode? Give it a hand!

Jerking off, wanking, hand jobbing, tossing, beating it, jacking, pulling cock or masturbating. Whatever we call it, masturbation is the way most of us first discover, in our early teens, the joys of orgasm.

Jerking off is not, however, confined to teenage years. Nor is it a mere forerunner to 'real' sex. It is a very satisfying way of cumming that most men rightly

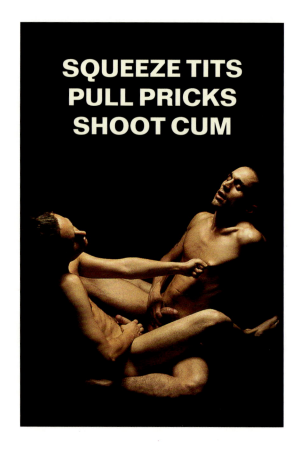

SQUEEZE TITS PULL PRICKS SHOOT CUM

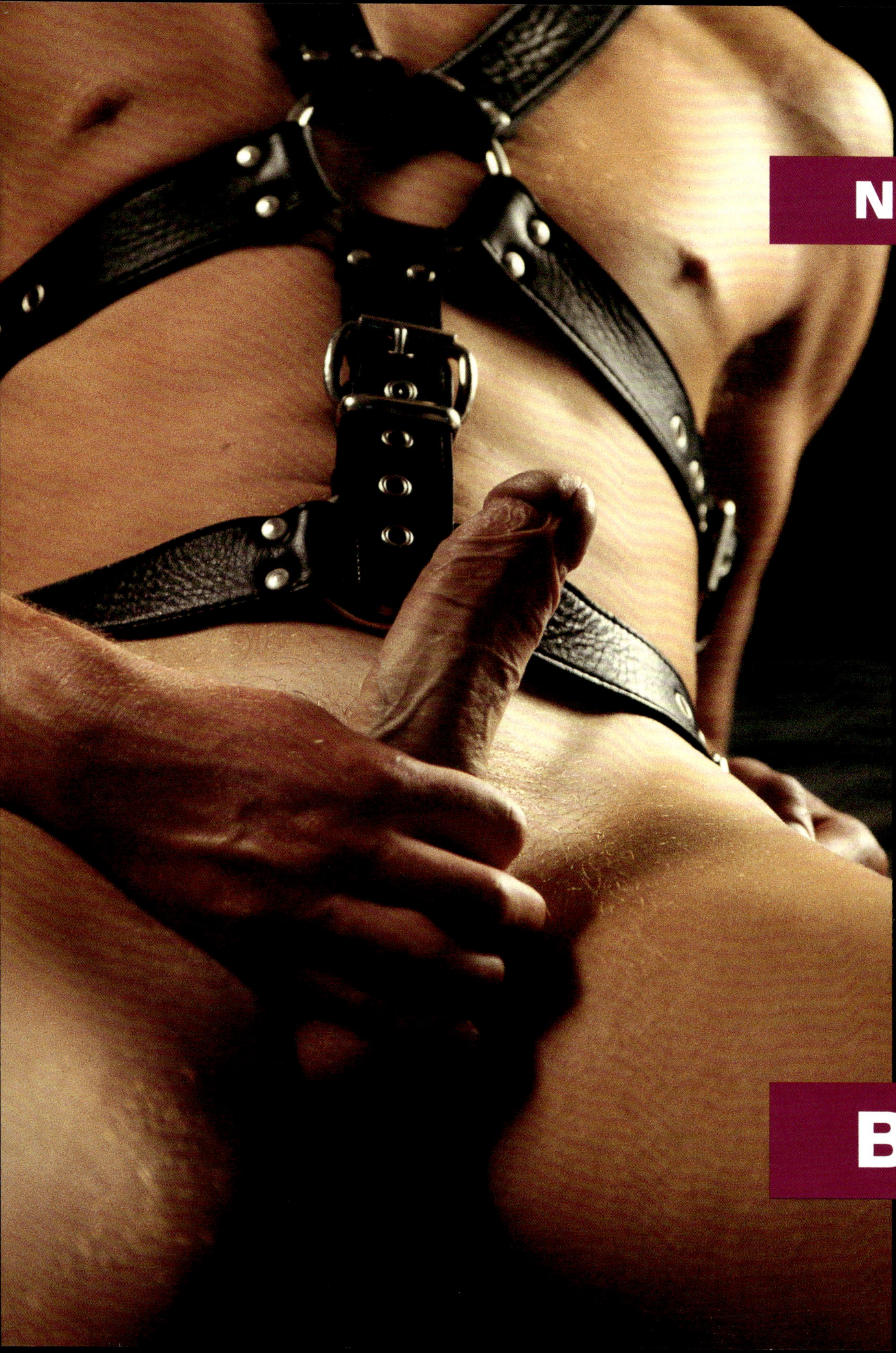

Cumming Together
Jerking off

NO RUBBER?

enjoy throughout their lives, whether they are single or in a relationship.

Even after experiencing sucking and fucking, many of us find we have some of our best orgasms when jerking off, either alone or with a partner. This is because when we wank ourselves we have total control over the momentum and rhythm of our climax. The constant feedback of sensations from our rampant prick to our brain allows us to instantly and accurately adjust our hand movements to get the best possible erotic feelings.

Jerking off alone is not necessarily a substitute for sex with another guy. Indeed, do-it-yourself orgasms have several advantages. You don't have to dress up, wine and dine him, make polite small talk, or put up with his snoring all night. It is sex without the complications of making it with someone else. Sometimes, that can be a pleasant relief.

However, guys who jerk off solo a lot can find it gets repetitive and dull. If that is your problem, stop jacking for a while to get yourself feeling hungry for sex. When you resume, vary your technique:

⚢ Hand fuck. Lubricate your fist and thrust into it with your cock. This shifts the focus of the motion from your hand to your pelvis and prick.

⚢ Bed fuck. Lie face down on the bed and rub your dick against the sheets, or against lubricated rubber if you prefer slippery, sliding raunchiness.

BEAT IT!

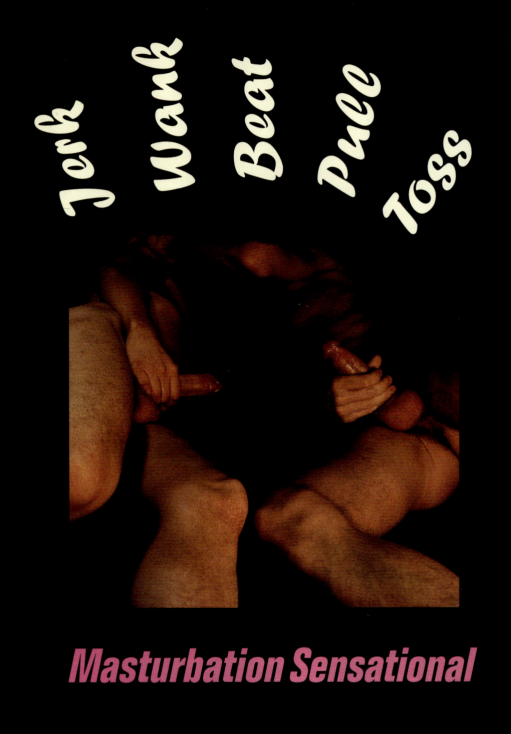

Jerk Wank Beat Pull Toss
Masturbation Sensational

✦ Use the hand opposite to the one you normally use to create the feeling of being played with by another man.

✦ Alternate between jerking off with and without lubricant, and experiment with different forms of lube to get different sensations.

✦ Dress up and act out your fantasies.

As well as doing it solo, jerking off can be a great way to cum with another guy. There are many different permutations. If you both like to have a lot of self-control over the action, you can wank yourself and your partner can wank himself. If you each prefer the thrill of a strange hand tossing your prick, you can jerk him and he can jerk you. Beating dick can be done simultaneously, or one after the other. Using both hands, you can do yourself and your partner at the same time. You can also jerk off another guy while being sucked by him, or wank yourself as he fucks you.

There are, furthermore, a variety of positions for mutual jerking off: both lying side by side, one lying on top of the other, both sitting up or standing up, and one lying down with the other sitting on top.

If your partner has difficulty wanking you in a way you enjoy, show him how you prefer it being done:

✦ Get him to put his hand loosely round your bulging cock.

✦ Then place your hand firmly over his.

✦ Now use his hand to jerk yourself off.

Safe jerking off

Jerking off is almost risk-free as there's no penetration. He cums on you, not in you. Your skin is like a giant all-over, natural condom. HIV cannot get through it. That means you can relax and enjoy having your man shoot his warm, wet cum onto your body. As the jets of spunk splash over you, grab his hand and use it to rub his cum all over your chest. Savour his luscious slurps as he licks his cum off your body.

The only risks are open wounds which break the flesh or severe skin disorders. The remedy is simple: cover them with a waterproof sticking plaster until they heal. If you use lubrication when jerking off, avoid using his cum to moisten your own dick; cum could get inside your piss-hole, and that might be dangerous.

Rubbing bodies

Cumming by rubbing bodies together is probably the most underrated way of having sex with another guy. It is incredibly safe. With no penetration, no cum gets inside the body. It can also, with skill and practice, be unbelievably erotic.

There are three main ways of achieving orgasm by rubbing bodies – belly rubbing, thigh rubbing and butt rubbing. Each have their own unique sensations.

Belly rubbing

This is rubbing your prick against another man's belly until you cum. You start by lying face-to-face with your partner. One of you lies on top of the other, or you both lie side by side, with your bodies pressed close together. If you like, put some lube on your cocks and bellies to create a smooth, slippery sexiness. Then rub your dick against your partner's stomach and cock, simulating the motion of fucking by moving your hips back and forth. Get him to do the same to you. Vary the pressure against his body, from firm lustful thrusts to light skin-skimming touches. Feel his iron-hard prick slap against your stomach. As you both get more and more aroused, thrust harder and faster until you climax, shooting cum over each other's bellies.

Belly rubbing is good for kissing because of the face-to-face position. There is a large area of mutual skin-against-skin body contact, which means all-over erotic stimulation from head to toe. It leaves both hands free for caressing, tit play, arse-fingering and massaging throughout the action.

Thigh rubbing

This involves rubbing your cock between a guy's legs to reach orgasm. Begin by getting your sex buddy to lie either face up or face down, with his legs crossed and his thighs held tightly together. Lube your dick and his legs. Then lower yourself on top of him. Push your prick between his thighs, and thrust backwards and forwards in a fucking-style movement.

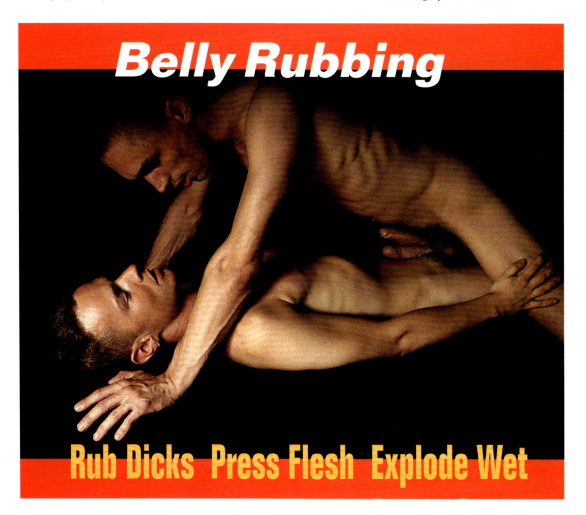

Belly Rubbing

Rub Dicks   Press Flesh   Explode Wet

Safer Sexy
Cumming Together

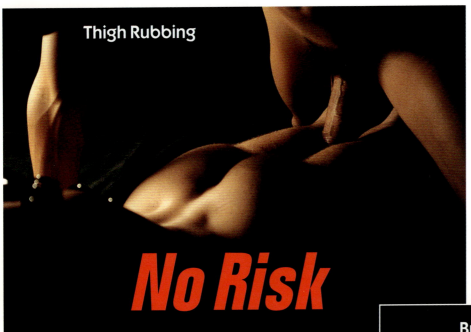
Thigh Rubbing — No Risk

Safe Rubbing

- If you have any visible cuts, cover them.

- If your dick is sore, it may be risky to get your partner's cum on it even if there are no wounds visible. Avoid getting his cum in your piss-hole.

- When thigh and butt rubbing, take care not to accidentally penetrate your partner's arse.

- If you are concerned about unintentionally slipping inside him, or if you think you might be tempted to switch from rubbing to fucking during the action, wear a condom when you thigh or butt rub.

- If you are the one being rubbed and cum gets near your arse-hole, make sure it doesn't get inside you. Wash your butt thoroughly.

Butt rubbing

This is rubbing your dick against a guy's butt until you climax, without penetrating his arse. Have your partner lie on his stomach. Grease his arse well, and press your body down on him. With strong pelvic movements, rub your dick horizontally to and fro between the cheeks of his arse. For variety, try butt rubbing with your partner lying face up on top of you, and you lying face up underneath him. From this position, with his body weight bearing down on you, there is a delicious feeling of being physically dominated and constrained. Butt rubbing from below also allows your partner to be jerked off at the same time as you rub his arse.

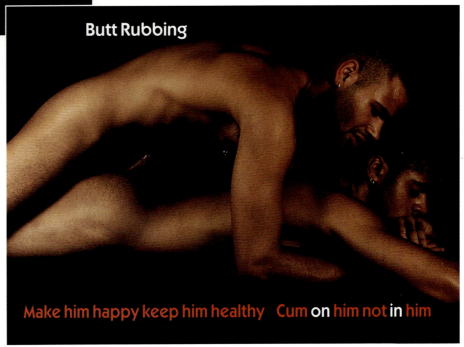
Butt Rubbing — Make him happy keep him healthy   Cum on him not in him

Sucking dick

Cock-sucking is also known as a blow job, giving head, oral sex and fellatio. The sexiness of sucking is its simplicity. Almost any position will do: standing or sitting up, kneeling or lying down. You don't even have to get undressed, which makes it ideal for a quickie in the bushes. Just unzip his fly and take his dick in your hand. Lick along its length. As his cock springs up hard, smother it in wet kisses. If he has a foreskin, gently ease it back. Using the tip of your tongue, circle the head of his cock and tickle his piss-hole.

Then, take his dick inside your mouth. Feel it swell up tight and taut as your lips engulf it in hot, moist flesh. Swallow him deep, until he bounces against the back of your throat. With your lips wrapped around his prick, slide up and down in long rhythmic movements. Wiggle your tongue along his cock as you go.

Vary the pressure of your lips, the intensity of your suction, and the pace of your head movements. Alternate between long, deep sucks and shorter, shallow ones. Every third or fourth time your lips slide down to the base of his dick, thrust your head hard to maximize penetration and nibble the base of his cock with your teeth.

For different sensations, try sucking his prick with a mouthful of hot water, ice-cubes, or peppermint tea.

Gagging

Deep-throat sucking is wickedly delicious, but it is an acquired skill. Initially, it often produces an involuntary gagging sensation, as if you are about to choke or vomit. Controlling this reflex reaction takes practice. The more dick you suck, the more your throat gets used to it. Some guys practise with a banana or dildo to help them overcome the retching sensation.

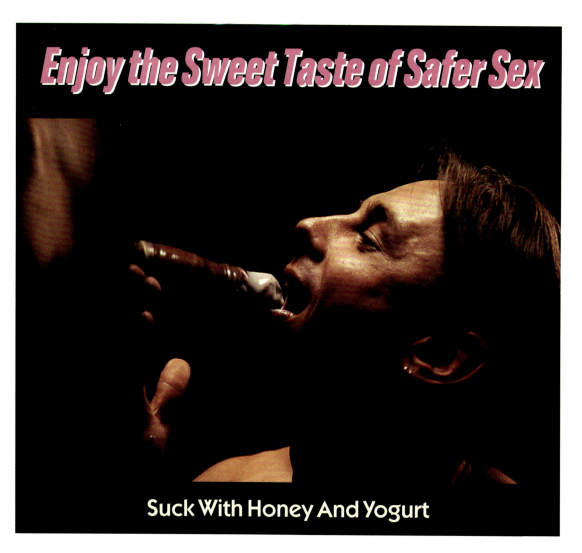

Big dick

If your man's cock is too big for you to swallow all the way without feeling choked, put your hand around the base of his shaft. This enables you to control the depth of his penetration. It also stimulates the base of his cock which your mouth cannot reach. As you get used to taking more of his dick in your mouth, gradually reduce your hand hold. Alternatively, try the sword-swallower's trick; lying on your back with your head hanging over the edge of the bed will straighten your throat and ease deeper dick penetration.

Cumming Together — **Safer Sexy**

Perverts in Paradise

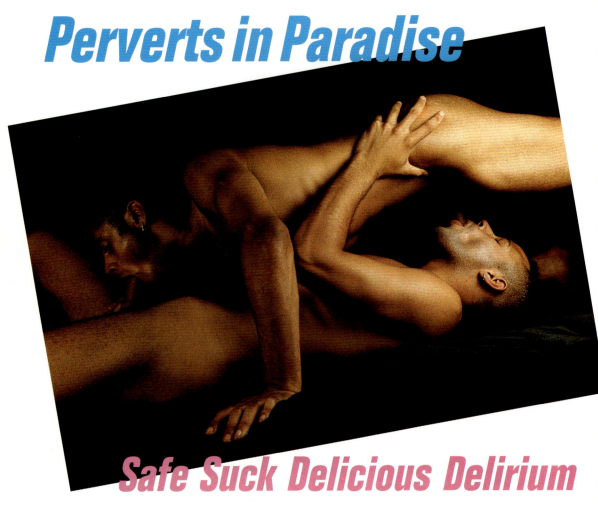

Safe Suck Delicious Delirium

Neckache

Sucking exercises muscles that rarely get used for anything else. If your neck gets tired, give it a rest. Let your hands do the work. Take his prick about halfway inside your mouth. Put your hand around the base of his cock and, keeping your head motionless, jerk him off into your mouth.

There are two other variations on sucking:

Mutual sucking

'69ing' is where both men suck off each other at the same time – lying side by side, or one on top and one below. This simultaneous sucking triggers reciprocal sexual frenzy. Each man gets added arousal from the slurping and stiffness of the other. '69' is especially good for guys who like to synchronize their sucking and cum together.

Face fucking

This is where the guy doing the sucking holds his mouth still while his partner thrusts his dick in and out. The movement is centred on the cock, not the lips. It means all the action is controlled by the guy being sucked. This enables him to adjust his position and momentum to get the best possible climax. Face fucking can also be a great turn on for guys who are into domination and degradation scenes. The person being sucked can be encouraged to constrain the head of the person doing the sucking in an arm lock while driving his prick into their mouth.

Safe sucking

Sucking is low-risk for HIV, and much safer than fucking without a condom. This is because it is harder to damage the inside of the mouth during sucking than the inside of the arse during fucking. The mouth is larger and less tight. HIV also tends to be inactivated by spit and stomach acids.

If sucking was a high-risk activity, a lot more gay men would have got HIV. According to medical records, only a small number of people are known to have caught the virus through sucking.

Although sucking is not 100% risk-free, the danger is very small. It is probably wise to avoid brushing your teeth just before sucking. This could cause tiny gum abrasions which, although not a major risk, may slightly increase your chances of HIV infection. Otherwise, providing your mouth is healthy, without any open wounds, sucking is no big danger. However, although the risk from getting cum or pre-

Cumming Together
Sucking dick

Clever Cocksuckers
Slurp Through Rubber

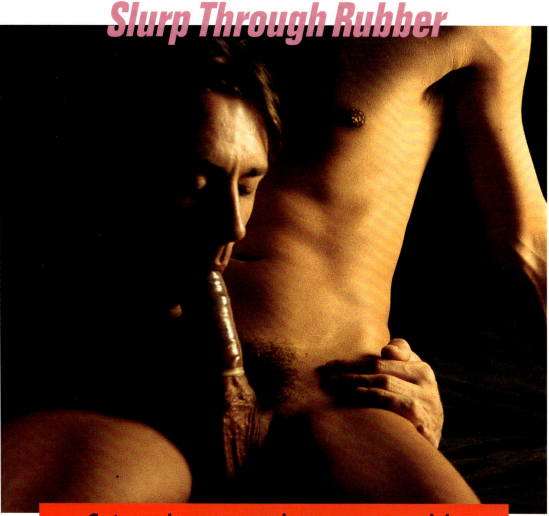

Cuts and sores may increase your risk. Otherwise, sucking is not a big danger for HIV

cum in the mouth is not great, some guys believe it is a risk not worth taking.

If you would rather be super-safe, get the guy you are sucking to pull his dick out of your mouth before he cums, or get him to wear a condom. A rubber will also help to protect you from other infections, such as gonorrhoea and syphilis, which can be transmitted by sucking. Be careful not to tear the rubber, or damage his cock, with your teeth.

Suck with a condom when you have cuts in your mouth, cracked lips, bleeding gums, cold sores, or a throat infection. Likewise, cover your suckmate's cock with a condom if it has scabs, redness, cuts, or a discharge.

Some guys choose unflavoured condoms because they get turned on by the taste of rubber or by the natural smell of a crotch. The only drawback is that many condoms are now pre-lubricated with spermicide, which is not very pleasant or healthy to lick. To overcome this problem, once the condom is rolled onto your partner's cock, gently wipe it with a clean handkerchief to remove the chemicals – or buy unlubricated rubbers.

Other men prefer flavoured condoms for sucking. They come in just about every flavour imaginable: banana, mint, cherry, mango, lemon and many more. It adds a whole new dimension to the slang expression 'suck a fruit'.

If you haven't got any flavoured condoms, improvise. When his dick is hard and he has put the condom on, raid the kitchen. Smear his condom-clad cock with jam, yoghurt, honey, or juice. Then, slurp away. Tasty!

Cumming Together — Safer Sexy

Fucking arse

Fucking, screwing, grinding, bumming, shagging, rogering, pumping or anal sex. Call it what you will, penetrating a guy's arse with your prick is glorious two-way pleasure.

The fucker gets enjoyment in his prick. The fuckee gets the thrill of having his prostate gland, deep inside his arse, massaged. There is also the psychological pleasure of penetration. Some guys like doing the screwing because of the sense of conquest and control it gives them. These feelings are not necessarily aggressive or domineering in a negative sense. They are often inspired by protective and bonding desires. Other men get off on the act of being screwed because it conjures up feelings of powerlessness and submission. Being physically overwhelmed and surrendering to penetration is an act of conscious vulnerability and trust which many guys find is a great sexual and emotional turn on. There is also a unique shared mental buzz from the act of fucking. Both partners, especially those in love, experience an intense emotional satisfaction from the sense of physical fusion and oneness.

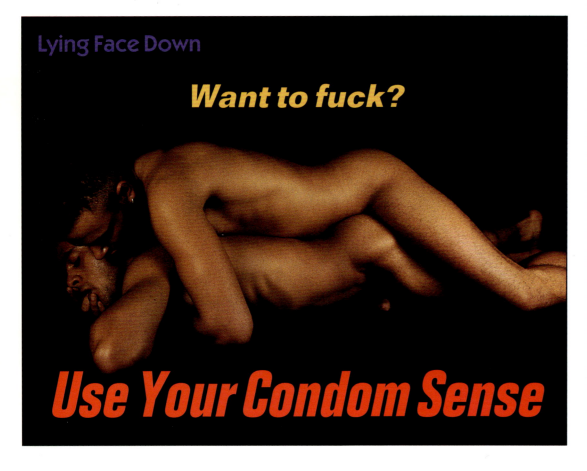

Lying Face Down — Want to fuck? Use Your Condom Sense

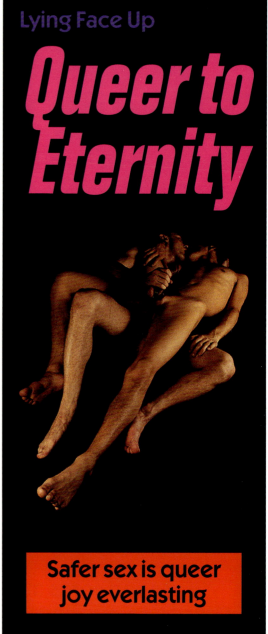

Lying Face Up — Queer to Eternity. Safer sex is queer joy everlasting

Cumming Together
Fucking arse

Lying Side by Side

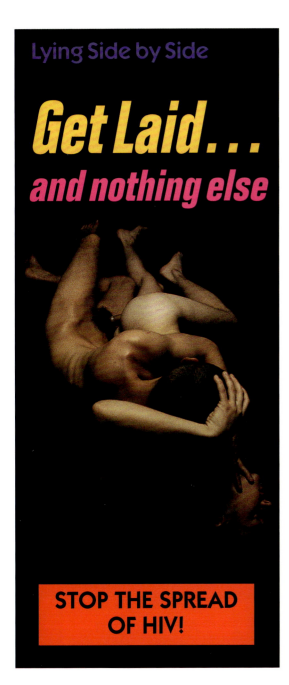

It is not, of course, always the man doing the screwing who is dominant. Sometimes, the guy being screwed is more in charge. This is the case with the 'sitting on it', 'sitting up together' and 'lying face up' positions. In these positions, the man who takes the dick inside him physically dominates his partner, and is also able to control the depth of penetration and the pace of thrusting. The penetrated partner is effectively doing the fucking because he is controlling the movement.

Most gay men are sexually versatile. They enjoy fucking and being fucked, and alternate between both roles. This ability to experience the dual dimensions of screwing is unique to gay sex. It is something straights can never know. That is their loss. Left with a one-sided experience of sex, they are often unable to understand and satisfy their partner. In contrast, one of the reasons gay men are so good at sex is because the majority of us are role-flexible. This means we know the ins and outs of giving and taking – what feels good and what does not. That makes us better at pleasing our partners, which is why we have such a high level of erotic satisfaction compared to straight men.

Kneeling upright

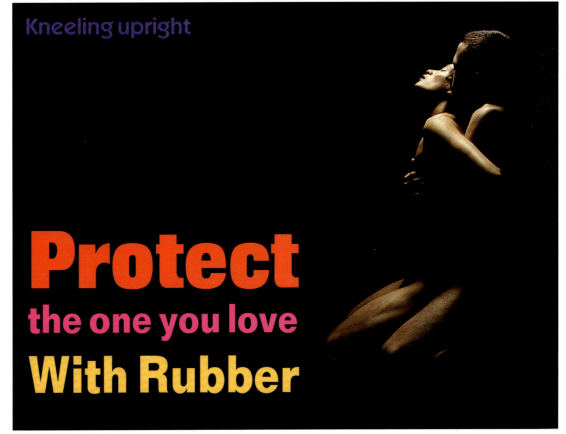

Cumming Together — Safer Sexy

On Hands & Knees

Get Off On Rubber

Cum Into Latex

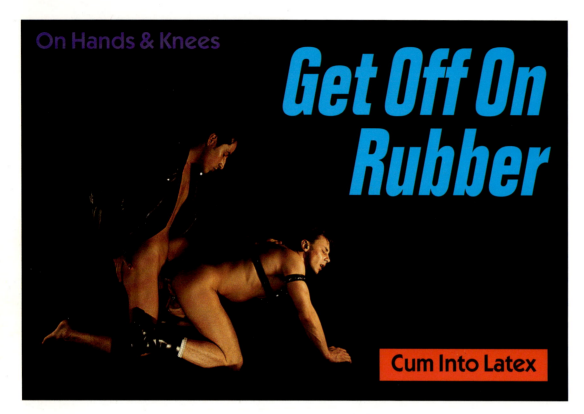

Standing Up

Fuck Men With HIV

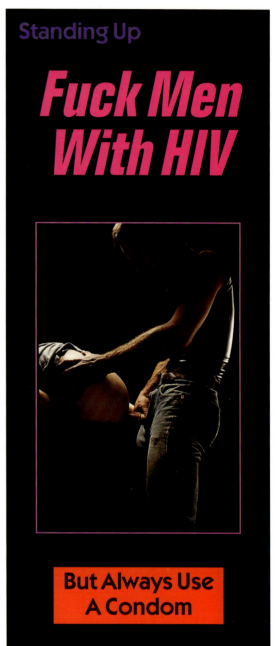

But Always Use A Condom

There are 13 basic positions for arse fucking – enough for a different position every day for a fortnight, with one day's rest. Each position involves different angles and depths of penetration, different points of body contact, and different erotic sensations. 'Face to face on top' and 'sitting up together face to face' allow for maximum depth of thrusting. 'Standing up' is especially suited to five-minute jobs in shop doorways and broom closets. 'On hands and knees' and 'lying face down' can embody elements of domination and submission. You can also improvise positions with the aid of household furniture. Try screwing in a rocking chair with your partner sitting on your prick. Or fuck on the kitchen table, with you standing and him lying with his legs in the air.

Every fuck should start by relaxing and arousing the guy who is going to be screwed. If you are the person doing the screwing, start by licking your partner's arse-hole with big wet slurps of your tongue. When he responds with twitching excitement, progress to fingering his butt. Try one finger to start with. Massage his prostate gland. As he gets more relaxed, add extra fingers to prise open his arse-hole.

Once you feel his muscles are relaxed, you will be raging with horniness. Now is the time to roll the condom on your dick and add some lube. Begin by pushing your prick softly against his opening. Use short, gentle, almost teasing, movements. Little-by-little increase the pressure on his hole. Only begin to penetrate him when you feel his arse-muscles open-

Face To Face On Top

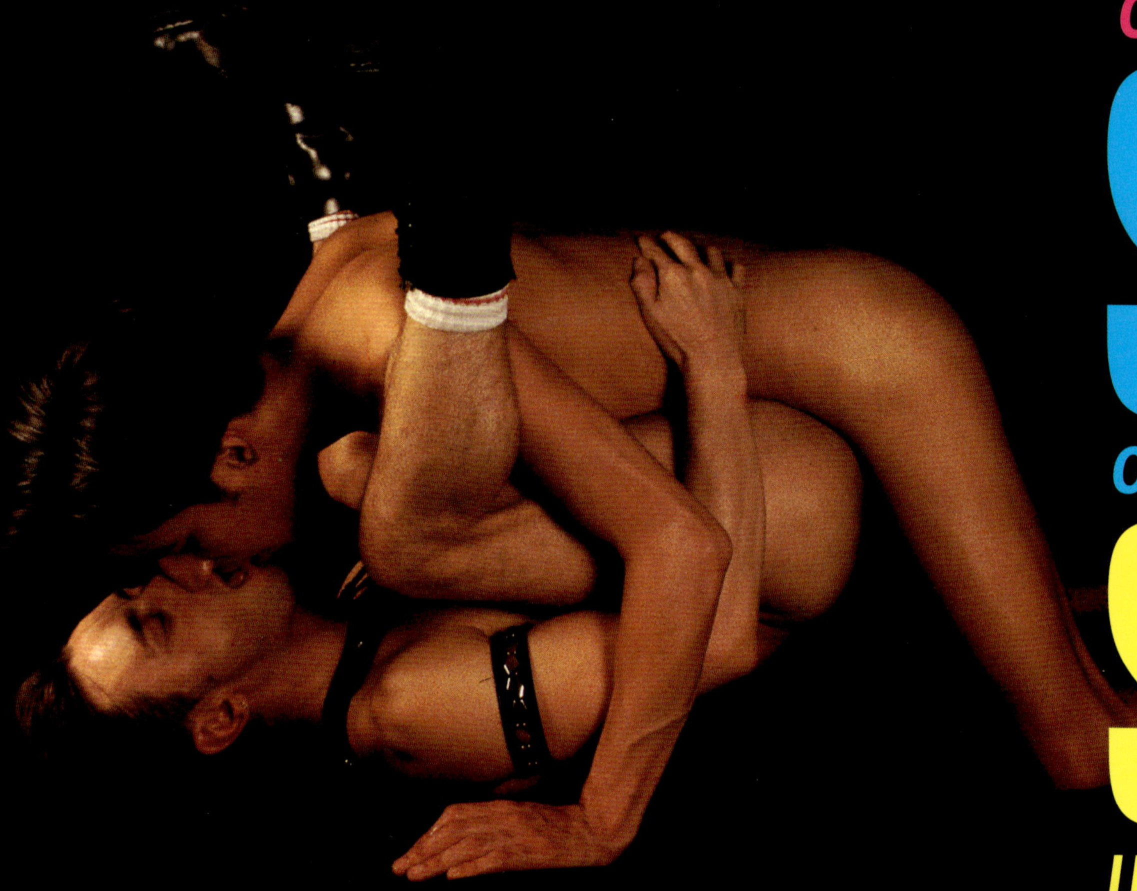

SLIP
ON A CONDOM
SLAP
ON SOME LUBE
SLAM
IN HIS ARSE-HOLE

53

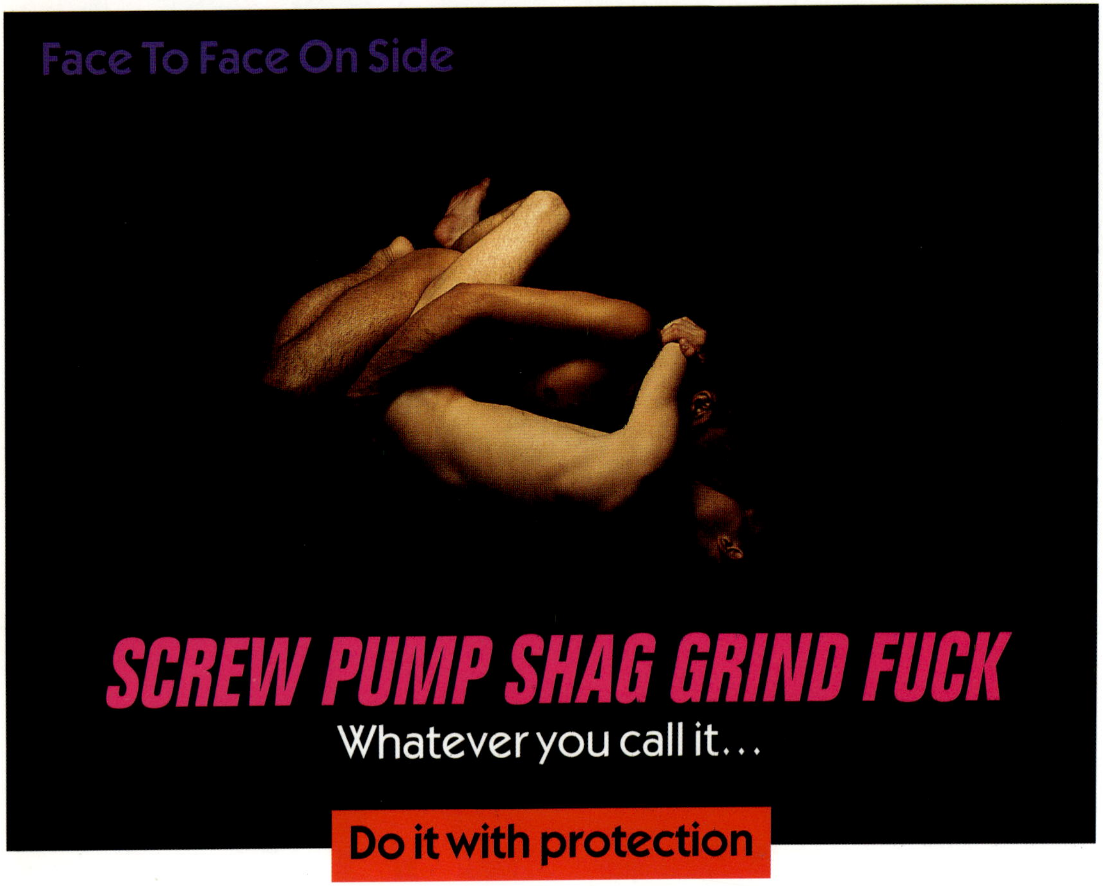

Safer Sexy
Cumming Together

Face To Face On Side

Face To Face Sideways Scissors

SCREW PUMP SHAG GRIND FUCK
Whatever you call it…

Do it with protection

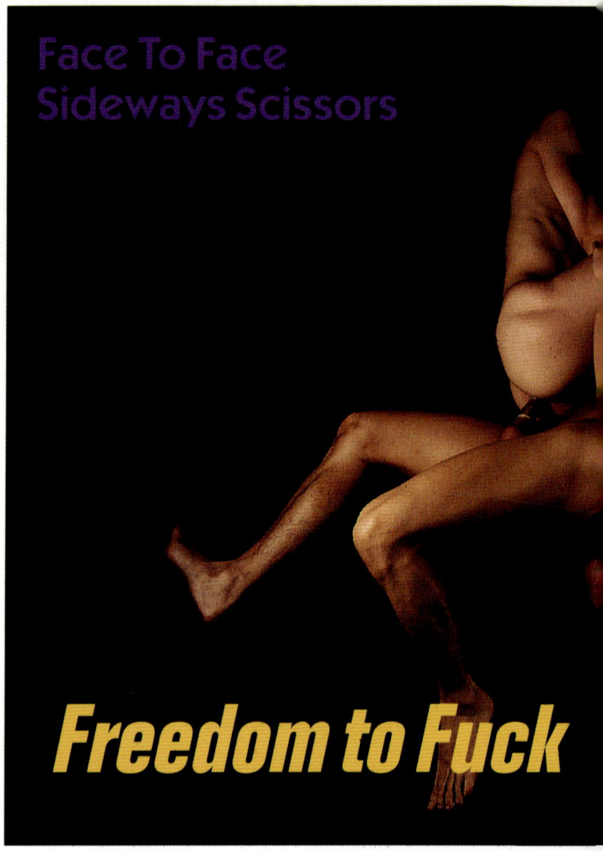

Freedom to Fuck

ing up to receive you. Enter him very slowly and gradually, with each forward thrust just a fraction deeper than the one before. Let his arse draw you inwards. When the head of your cock is inside him, pause for a minute to allow him to get accustomed to it. During this pause, jerk his dick to arouse and relax him. This will ease penetration. If your partner's butt feels tense and tight, do not force your prick inside. That could cause him pain. If he feels pain, he will probably want to stop fucking and both of you will lose out. You won't get to fuck him, and he won't get to enjoy the delights of being screwed.

A forced fuck could also tear the lining of his arse – risking loss of blood, serious infection, and dangerous complications. Whenever you notice signs of blood during fucking, stop immediately. Apart from the possibility of serious damage to the arse, blood can contain highly infectious concentrations of HIV and hepatitis B.

If the guy you are screwing experiences pain, slowly withdraw your cock and allow the discomfort to subside. Playfully caress the outside of his arse-hole with your fingers. Very gradually work them inside him again, gently massaging his butt muscles as you go. When you have got them relaxed, you can try to penetrate him once more with your prick. Ever so carefully, extend yourself deeper into him.

If he feels discomfort at this stage, it may be due to trapped wind. He should have a good fart. Pain could also be caused by your thrusting from an uncomfortable angle. Try pointing your prick in a different direction. Or it might be because your cock is too big for him. Choose a position which restricts your depth of penetration, such as 'lying side by side', or wrap your fist around the base of your cock to stop yourself going in so deep.

Cumming Together
Fucking arse

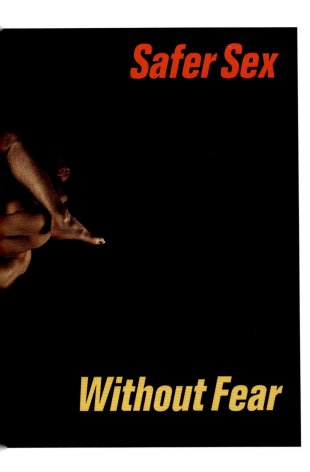

Safer Sex

Without Fear

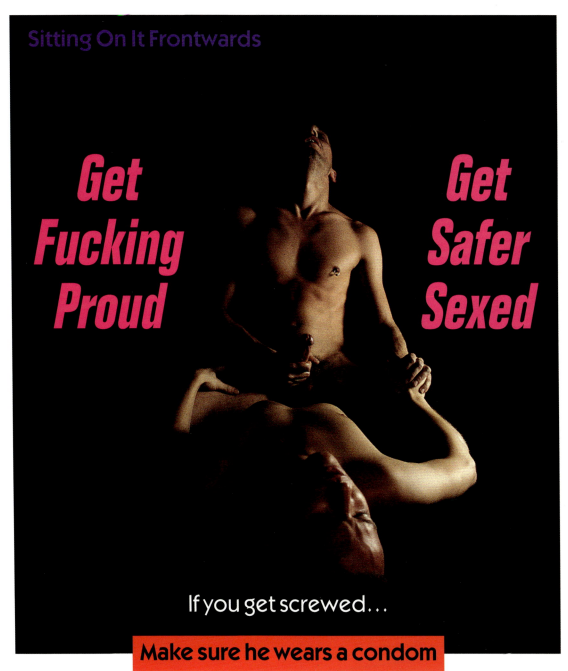

Sitting On It Frontwards

Get Fucking Proud

Get Safer Sexed

If you get screwed…

Make sure he wears a condom

When you are sure your partner is fully relaxed and comfortable, you can pump and grind to your dick's delight. Slide in and out of his slippery, silky arse-hole with long, strong thrusts. Feel his pulsing butt muscles clench around your shaft in spasms of erotic relish. Ram your rigid prick deep into his guts, right up to the hilt. Press your balls and pubic hair hard against his wet hole. Hold the pressure. Writhe and wriggle, using your whole body weight, to edge your cock inside him that extra fraction further to produce sheer body-shuddering pleasure. Push. Squeeze. Kiss. Bite. Scream.

Safer Sexy
Cumming Together

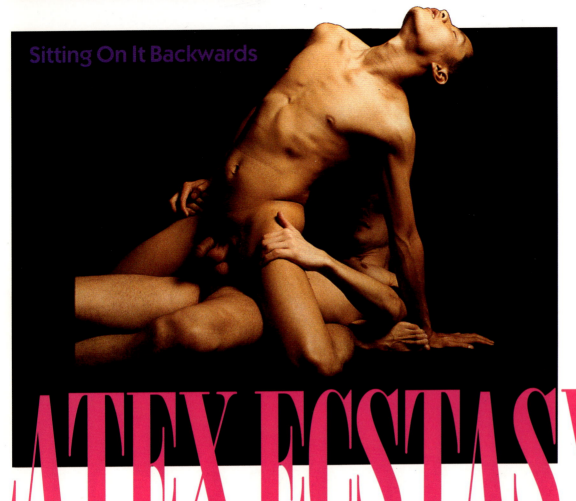

Sitting On It Backwards

LATEX ECSTASY

heaving, sweating. Forget all your inhibitions. Let your bodies go. Thrash around in wild uncontrollable lust. As you both reach the crescendo of orgasm, feel his arse muscles throb and contract around your cock. Feel your prick stretch tight to bursting point as bolts of indescribable pleasure shoot along its length. As you explode, with jet after jet of warm spunk, release all your sexual energy in screams of rapture.

Once you have cum, rest in each other's arms for a moment to enjoy the after-glow. But do not leave it too long. Before you go limp, slowly withdraw your cock. Hold the base of the condom to stop it slipping off. Do not pull out fast, as this could cause your partner pain. When you are fully withdrawn, remove the rubber, tie a knot in the end, and wrap it in tissue. Wipe the cum off your cock. Then relax with your partner. Hug, caress and kiss each other.

HIV and other infections can survive for some hours outside the body. If you plan to have sex again later, it is sensible to take a shower or bath before any repeat performance.

First Time

Initially, many of us find being screwed uncomfortable, even painful. This is because our arse muscles are naturally tight. Their principal function is to hold in shit until we are ready to crap. It takes time and effort to unlearn this natural reflex in order to get the arse to relax sufficiently to enjoy a good screwing.

It helps if, before you first get fucked, you have spent some time alone exploring your arse-hole with your fingers or a dildo. This will loosen and relax your arse muscles. When you decide you are ready to be screwed, choose a partner who is sensitive and patient – not just anyone. Make sure he has experience of being fucked himself. That way he will understand what it's like, and be better able to help you overcome any fears or discomfort.

If you are close to climax but don't want to cum yet, take a breather. Rest your dick inside your partner for a couple of minutes. Just lie there, kissing and caressing him all over. Check the condom hasn't broken. Tickle his arse with your fingers while you examine it. If the rubber is still in one piece, slip back inside him. But this time, let your partner do all the action. Have him push his steamy arse-hole against you, burying your dick in his hot flesh. As you swell up inside him, stiffer than ever, stroke his towering prick. Squeeze him gently to milk out his pre-cum. Rub it over his shaft. Then grasp his cock firmly and begin to jerk him off. Rock your bodies together in rhythmic motion. Synchronize the plunges of your prick with the strokes of your hand. Listen to his breathing and observe his muscle contractions to coordinate your build up to climax.

Inhale the sexy smells of his crotch. Turn on to the sounds of your dick splashing in and out of his juicy arse. Quicken the pace to fever-pitch – gasping,

Cumming Together
Fucking arse

Pain when being fucked

The most common reason men don't enjoy being screwed is psychological – fear, nervousness, and tension. The result: their arse muscles are tight and it hurts them to get fucked. If you are not used to being screwed, or find it uncomfortable, the most important thing is to learn to relax:

- Loosen your arse-hole with your fingers.
- Take long, slow, deep breaths.

The guy screwing you must not rush sex. That will only increase your anxiety and tension. He should spend a lot of time licking and fingering your butt before attempting to enter you. It's also a good idea for him to jerk you off as he begins to penetrate you. This will get you turned on, helping you to relax and building up an association in your mind between penetration and pleasure.

It's easier if you choose a sexual position which is less likely to cause pain. 'Lying side by side' limits the depth of penetration, and 'sitting on it' enables the person being fucked to control the action. Discomfort when he enters you will also be reduced by pushing your butt muscles outwards (as if you were about to have a shit). This opens up your arse-hole and makes it easier for his dick to slide inside. If his cock is too big for comfort, hold your hand around the base of his dick to limit his penetration to a depth you can cope with.

Constipation

A constipated arse is not very sexy if you want to finger or fuck. A longterm solution: switch to a high-fibre diet to ensure regular, well-formed shits that leave your arse clean and empty. The immediate solution: take a crap if you plan to be screwed. Although not recommended for everyday use, you can also try washing out your arse with a douche, or enema. These consist of a small plastic or rubber bag with a nozzle. After filling the bag with warm water, the nozzle is inserted into the butt. The bag is squeezed, and the water squirts inside. The water is then shitted into the toilet. This gets rid of any shit, leaving the arse empty and screwable. Don't forget, if you use a douche or enema, never share it with your partner, as this could spread infection.

Sitting Up Together Face To Face

BUTTFUCKERS

Condom Lovers

Cumming Together — Safer Sexy

Sitting Up Together From Behind

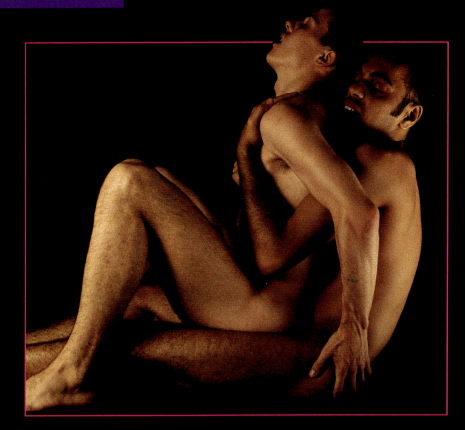

Love Yourself
Love Each Other
Love Safe

Safe fucking

Fucking arse without a condom is very high risk for HIV and other sexually-transmitted diseases. *It's by far the most risky sexual act*. The vast majority of men with HIV got it from screwing without a rubber – either from being screwed or from doing the screwing. The virus can pass both ways when two men fuck. If you are being fucked, HIV can infect you through the lining of your arse. If you are fucking, HIV can enter through the opening of your dick-hole or through scratches on your cock which can be so tiny you may not be able to see or feel them. Many men who only fuck – but never get fucked – have contracted the virus in this way. If there is only one safer sex rule you always stick to, make sure it is this: *never fuck arse without a condom*.

Getting your partner to pull out his dick before he cums is no protection, either for you or for him. Pre-cum can contain HIV and get into your butt. Arse juices, especially if they are contaminated with blood, can contain HIV and enter his piss-hole. Using a douche or enema to wash out your arse after screwing without a condom won't protect you against HIV. In fact, it will probably spread the virus around inside you and may even increase your likelihood of infection.

Wearing a rubber massively reduces the risk of HIV when you fuck. It cuts the risk to both partners to negligible proportions. Condoms are not, however, totally safe. A very small percentage have holes. Others have faults which cause them to break. Sometimes, they disintegrate because an oil-based lubricant was used, or they slip off in the passion of the screwing.

When fucking, remember:

⚭ Choose an extra strong brand of condom which carries a safety standard logo and an expiry date.

⚭ Use lots of water-based lube – not oil.

⚭ During the fuck, check regularly to make sure the rubber is still on and has not broken.

Happy screwing!

Diversity and Spice
Love and let love

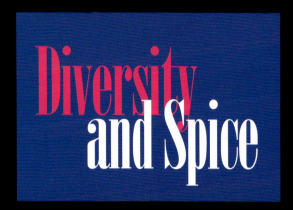

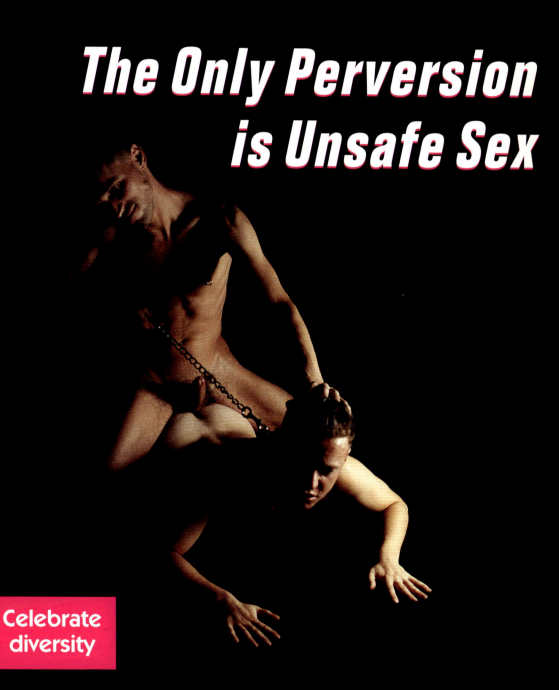

The Only Perversion is Unsafe Sex

Love and let love

Human sexuality embraces a glorious diversity of feelings, emotions, desires and attractions. We are all unique individuals with our own unique erotic tastes. We get sexually aroused and fulfilled in a huge variety of different ways. Many of these ways are familiar and accepted. Others, such as piercing and sadomasochism (SM), may seem strange and even unpleasant to some people. However sexual difference is part of the spice of life. One man's sexual nightmare is another man's sexual heaven.

You may not be turned on by a particular sexual act, but others are. Sex play with piss and shit is very much a minority interest but that doesn't make it wrong. Guys who get pleasure from it feel it is right for them, and that's justification enough. Providing sex is mutually safe, *freely* agreed by all participants, satisfying and harmless, no one has a right to condemn what others do in bed.

Nevertheless, there are plenty of moralists who want to control our sexuality. Fearful of diversity, they use terms like 'normality' and 'abnormality' to validate their own prejudices and marginalize anything out of the ordinary. Only the dull and the dead never deviate from the sexual norm. Sexual deviance is any desire that differs from what moralists consider

Celebrate diversity

Diversity and Spice — Safer Sexy

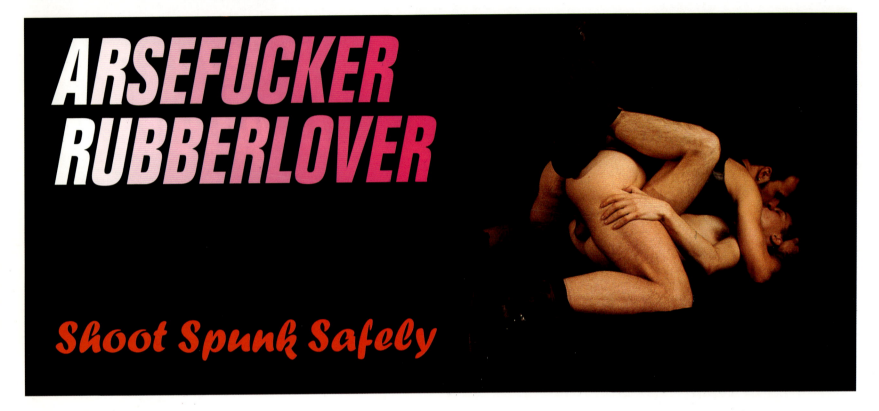

ARSEFUCKER RUBBERLOVER

Shoot Spunk Safely

to be normal. But the difference between 'normality' and 'deviance' is precarious. Most of us like love-bites. But is a hard love-bite far removed from sado-masochism? A playful slap may be considered a spanking by some. But how different are they? 'Deviance' is often, it seems, nothing more than a stronger version of 'normal' sex.

Putting moral judgements aside, what some people call 'deviance' is just a specialized sexual taste. It involves reaching orgasm in ways that are different from familiar ways. For example, corporal punishment or sex over the phone may be considered unusual or exotic by some people, but that doesn't mean they're bad.

There is no obligation for any of us to join in sexual acts we don't enjoy, but it is good to be open to new erotic experiences. Unless we try things, how can we be certain whether we like them or not? There's no harm in experimenting. If new activities don't turn us on, we don't have to do them again. On the other hand, we might discover that not only are most so-called 'perversions' harmless, some of them are a lot of fun.

Too many of us limit our sexual repertoire because of ignorance, prejudice, fear, or sheer lack of imagination. The full potential of our libido remains unexplored. The result can be a narrow and conventional sex life. There are those of us, of course, who are completely satisfied with a basic sexual menu. But some of us get bored and our erotic appetites need reviving with diversity.

Don't be put off exploring sexual acts that others label perverse. A 'perversion' is the label people give to any sexual act they themselves don't enjoy. This judgemental attitude is usually a reflection of their personal hang-ups. Were the truth to be known, most of us are excited by some form of sex that someone else would call perverse.

Deviate and celebrate! The only kind of sex to definately avoid is unsafe sex, and sex without mutual consent and fulfilment. Otherwise, anything goes. It's up to you to make your own choices about the kind of sex you want. Whatever you decide, respect the sexual differences of others, even if you don't share them. Love and let love.

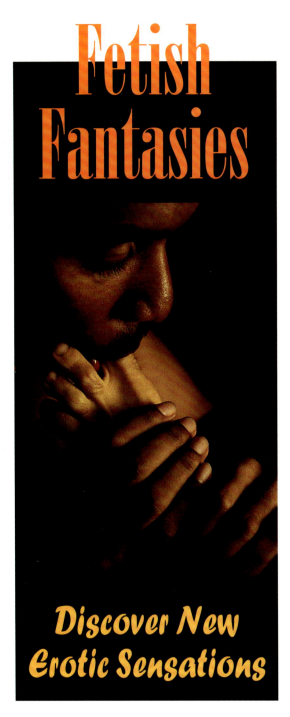

Fetish Fantasies
Discover New Erotic Sensations

Diversity and Spice
Fetishes and fixations

Fetishes and fixations

Sexual attraction is not innate. The kind of guy that makes us stiff and sticky is partly a result of personal experience. This experience includes our male role-models during childhood, the type of guys we first had sex with, our men friends and acquaintances in adult life. Sexual attraction is also very significantly influenced by the cultural images of maleness projected by movies, fashion and pop music. As a result, who we find sexually attractive is often culturally-specific, and tends to change over time. Muscles, long hair, leather, moustaches, suntans, piercings and androgyny may be fashionable in one culture and not in another, in one decade and not in the next. These combined influences of individual experiences and cultural values mean that we are generally attracted to certain types of bodies more than to others. We get turned on by guys of a specific physical shape, build, height or colour. We also tend to get aroused by particular parts of the body. Many of us drool over a square jaw-line, hairy chest, bulging biceps, pinched waist, or circumcized cock.

All these attractions are different forms of fetishism. A fetish is anything non-sexual which produces sexual arousal. PVC vests and leather jackets, for instance, are not sexual in themselves. However, lots of men find them very horny. Likewise, there is nothing intrinsically erotic about toes and feet. Yet toe-sucking and foot-licking is the height of sensuality for some guys. There are a lot of different and complex reasons why people develop fetishes. Many fetish attractions result from experiences where an object, perhaps a pair of boxer shorts or a nipple ring, becomes associated with very strong and memorable sexual excitement. As a result, that object gets eroticized in the mind and thereafter stimulates sexual arousal.

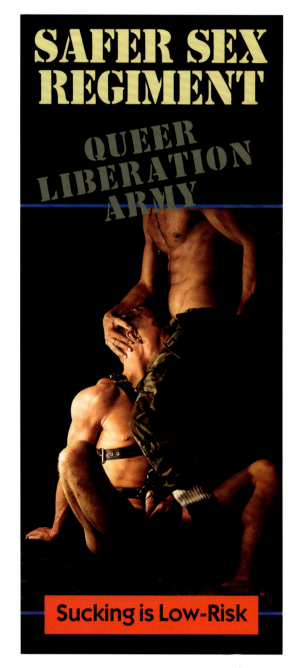

SAFER SEX REGIMENT
QUEER LIBERATION ARMY

Sucking is Low-Risk

Diversity and Spice — Safer Sexy

Divine Deviants
Choose Life Love Safe

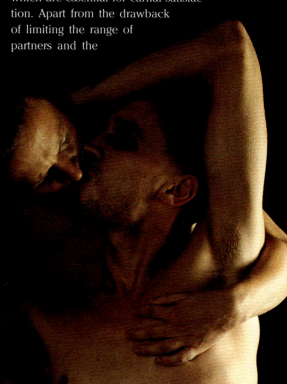

Fetishism covers many different types of attraction:

- *Physique* – chubby, tall, beefcake, stocky, thin.
- *Body parts* – thighs, feet, tits, nose, arse, hands.
- *Clothing* – white socks, dirty underwear, DM boots.
- *Adornments* – stubble, earrings, crewcut, tattoos, beard.
- *Personality* – intelligence, warmth, humour, shyness.
- *Body language* – hand gestures, walk, smile, posture.
- *Locations* – shower, alleyway, armchair, forest, toilet, locker room.
- *Tastes and smells* – sweat, chocolate, cock cheese, aftershave.

Some fetishes are fairly exotic like being tied up with lace briefs, giving enemas, and dressing up in nappies or gas masks. However, most fetishes are not too dissimilar from ordinary forms of attraction. Some, such as torn blue jeans, are little more than highly sexualized versions of everyday fashions. This begs the question: at what point does a pair of Levi 501s cease to be a sexy fashion accessory and become a fetish object? The distinction is ambiguous, and this suggests that fetishes are often not very different from mainstream desires.

A lot of common fetishes relate to styles of clothing which variously project images of masculinity, power, athleticism, sexiness or androgyny:

- Leather jackets, denim jeans, check flannel shirts and work boots evoke maleness, strength, potency and toughness.
- Military, police, security guard and firefighter uniforms conjure associations with authority, power and discipline.
- Jockstraps, track suits, sweat bands and trainers imply physical stamina, muscularity, health, fitness and sporting prowess.
- Lycra shorts, string vests, rubber one-pieces and leather briefs have connotations of sexual availability and unbridled lust.
- Floral shirts, silk underwear, cashmere pullovers and satin trousers suggest softness, refinement and gender ambiguity.

Of all the many different gay fetishes, those revolving around masculinity are the most pervasive. In recent decades the dominant gay icons have been the body builder, cowboy, motorbiker, lumberjack, construction worker and soldier. Machismo has become synonymous with queerness. This appropriation of straight male images is also profoundly subversive.

What gay men have done is transform and re-invent traditional masculinity. While retaining and even magnifying the macho style, we have discarded its aggression and rendered it non-threatening. Queer masculinity embodies the eroticism of maleness without the menace of heterosexual machismo. It is the triumph of style over pathology.

Whatever our sexual tastes, a majority of us enjoy some kind of fetish. These fetishes are not perverse, just different. Some may be unusual, but that does not mean they merit disapproval. What repels one of us can be very attractive to another. Providing there is no coercion or exploitation, fetishes do no harm and can make sex much more interesting.

For some men, fetishes are preferences they enjoy but can do without. For others, they are fixations which are essential for carnal satisfaction. Apart from the drawback of limiting the range of partners and the opportunities for sex, there is nothing to be said against fetish fixations. Many men get great pleasure from them. You can too. It's your choice.

Threesomes and orgies

Two men is company. Three is a crowd. Four or more is an orgy of queer desire. Getting screwed by one guy while you fuck a second guy, suck a third guy, and jerk off a forth guy is an electrifying (and delightfully exhausting) erotic experience. For brain teasing types, it can also be a fascinating jigsaw-style puzzle to work out all the possible combinations of pricks and orifices. Four men can be arranged in dozens of permutations of sucking, jerking and screwing.

For men in longterm relationships, there is the perennial problem of how to survive the sexual routine which, after a couple of years, can begin to dull even the most committed partnership. If you don't like the idea of your lover going off by himself with another guy, threesomes offer a less threatening option – you can both enjoy sex with other men in circumstances where you share the experience. Some couples find this strengthens the trust and bond between them, as well as revivifying their sex lives.

Stripping off and having sex in front of other guys can help overcome inhibitions and hang-ups, such as body shyness and sexual guilt. Sex with a group can also be a fun way to learn new sexual tricks and treats fast; but be aware that gay orgies are illegal in some countries.

Safe orgies

Orgies involve having sex simultaneously with several men, and usually cumming more than once. This can increase the possibility of passing infectious body fluids between partners. Even if you use a new condom every time, fucking one guy after

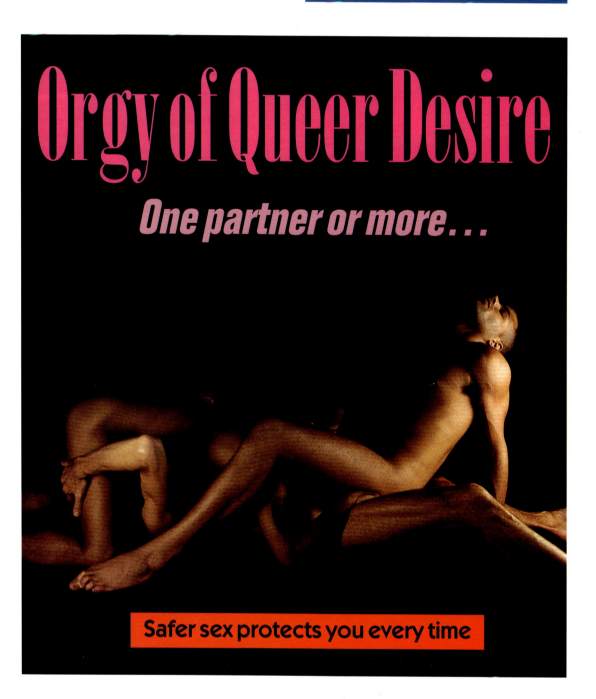

another may involve a slight risk. Cum, blood or shit from your just-used condom could get on your hands as you roll it off, and then be transferred from your hands to a new condom as you roll it on. Once on a new condom, the infectious fluid can pass easily into the arse of the next man as you sink your prick inside him. Similarly, screwing and fingering can spread shit and arse juices, and licking the bum of a man who has been screwed moments beforehand could result in the contraction of various arse-borne diseases. Orgies are not, however, inherently dangerous, as long as you take care. If you want to err on the side of caution, you can reduce the risks of orgies by mutually arranging to restrict the action to jerking off only. Alternatively, you may agree to fuck, but suggest that everyone showers after each orgasm.

Dirty sex

Some men hate fresh-scrubbed and sweet-smelling sex. It strikes them as unnatural, contrived and unerotic. Their strongest arousal comes from ripe unwashed bodies, dirty clothes and filthy surroundings. They see these as embodying a raw, hard-edged, untamed masculinity and lust. These qualities also often attract them to tough and aggressive men, such as skinheads, Hell's Angels, soldiers and truckers.

Guys into sleaze revel in the pungent odours and tastes of sweaty armpits, greasy skin, cheesy cock, smelly feet, shitty arse and oily hair. Their libido goes into overdrive at the sight and smell of a man wearing grimy jeans, a sweat-wet T-shirt, day-old stubble, and cum-stained boxer shorts. Poking their prick up a filthy, stinking arse-hole in a car mechanic's workshop, piss-soaked doorway, muddy construction site or shit-splattered toilet cubicle is absolute bliss.

Safe dirt

Dirty sex is very low-risk for HIV but it may be more risky for infections like hepatitis A and B and gut parasites. These infections can be contracted when body fluids get spread around and are not cleaned up after sex.

Anonymous quickies

Sexual enjoyment can be had, if desired, without emotional commitment or 'getting to know you'. That's what spontaneous, quick and anonymous sex in parks, toilets, saunas and backrooms is all about: sexual release and nothing else. You see what you want, get hard, and go for it. No questions asked. No justifications expected. All that is required is momentary mutual pleasure.

Some men find this kind of sex very honest and liberating. It's straightforward and direct, with no pretence or prevarication. There's a strong streak of egalitarianism about it: in darkness and shadows, youth or good looks count for less. Because partners don't get to know each other first, quick sex tends to be a classless melting pot. Bankers do it with brickies. All are part of the same community of cocks seeking the same lustful release. This no-strings sexual exchange is also ideal for men in committed partnerships who need occasional sexual escape but who want to remain emotionally loyal to their partner.

Uncomplicated and demanding nothing more than shared lust, anonymous sex has its own unique thrills. Sharing bodies with a total stranger involves an exhilarating combination of risk and trust. Curiosity and nervous apprehension mix with sexual anticipation and horniness. The fantasy of the unknown and the excitement of the new are powerful erotic stimulants. Added to these is the frisson of danger that accompanies anonymous sex in an eerie location like a deserted park in the middle of the night.

Contrary to the idea that quick sex is invariably impersonal and emotionless, it isn't always. Tenderness is not the exclusive prerogative of guys in relationships. Fucking a man you met only minutes before can embody elements of romance and affection. Indeed, one-off encounters are often incredibly passionate and intense, precisely because of their never-to-be-repeated nature. They may be even partly spurred by feelings or fantasies of affection as much as by raw libido. Sometimes, what starts out as anonymous sex can lead to an exchange of phone numbers and develop into a longterm love affair.

Safe quickies

Anonymous sex is often in locations where there is a danger of being caught, such as parks and toilets. Those involved therefore tend to avoid fucking which, with your trousers around your ankles, makes a fast get-away difficult. They usually stick to jerking and sucking which enable cocks to be quickly zipped out of sight. Most quickies are thus very low risk for HIV; although they may involve a risk of arrest.

Porn

Gay pornography makes visible and explicit the homoerotic desires that society wants to deny and suppress. It's a positive affirmation of gayness which presents homosexuality as something arousing and pleasurable. No wonder that homophobes find it so threatening, and we find it so appealing. In a hetero-centric society, gay pornography is sexually subversive and homo-empowering. Its explicit images of queer sexuality validate our erotic feelings and scorn

Diversity and Spice
Sex over the phone

Roll 'N' Ride

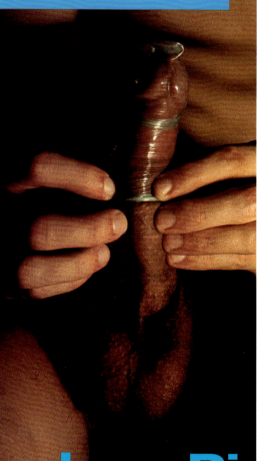

straight hang-ups. The defiant parade of male flesh pressed against male flesh is an in-your-face challenge to the cultural hegemony of heterosexuality.

Homo pornography is an honest representation of the male body in various states of undress and sexual action. Since there is nothing wrong with nudity and sex between men, visual images of that nudity and sex cannot be wrong. Only a body-hating, sex-phobic and anti-gay culture resorts to censorship of queer love and lust.

Porn videos, drawings, photographs and stories can be helpful sex aids which enhance erotic skills and satisfaction. For some men they act as a de facto form of gay sex education, giving graphic and no-holds-barred tips on erotic techniques. They can also provide a safety valve for unfulfilled and frustrated desires, and allow the exploration of sexual fantasies, including dangerous ones, without putting anyone at risk.

For men who have been lovers for many years, watching porn videos as a prelude to sex can help sustain erotic enthrallment and prevent a relationship from losing its sexual sparkle. Others who find it difficult to meet sexual partners because they live in isolated communities, sometimes find that porn is one of their few means of sexual fulfilment.

The only drawback about porn is that it may encourage unrealistic expectations from real-life sexual partners. If you have been jerking off to video images of beefcake hunks who cum six times an hour, the guys you meet in your local bar may seem rather tame by comparison. But even the most ordinary real life partner has a physical warmth and interactive capacity that the best porn stars lack!

Safe porn

Using porn as an aid to jerking off is a totally safe form of sex, which can help reduce the spread of HIV. No partner, absolutely no risk!

Sex over the phone

Jerking off while talking dirty with a guy on the telephone is another completely risk-free safer sex option. It can be done with a friend you know, a lover who is away from home on a work assignment, or with someone anonymous contacted via a phone sex line or magazine advert.

Not knowing the person you are speaking to can be especially exciting because you can form your own mental image, and project on to him your most brazen fantasies. It is, of course, also very egalitarian. It doesn't matter what you look like, how you dress, or how old you are. All that counts is what you sound like. Furthermore, dialling a sex line or a personal ad number is completely anonymous and means no obligations or commitments. This tends to loosen inhibitions; it can make coping with rejection much easier.

Roll on a Condom   Ride Him Wild

Safer Sexy
Diversity and Spice

Phone sex is one occasion when it is okay to lie. Check out what kind of guy your phone partner likes, then give him an image of yourself similar to his tastes. If he wants nine inches of thick prime beef thrust down his throat, let him have it (even if you are really a standard six inches). That way, you will fulfil his cravings and give him a great orgasm. He'll want to come back to you for more.

Since all the thrills of sex over the phone are based on noise, be sure to make lots of filthy loud sounds. Talk about your voluptuous, purple-red, towering cock. Breathe heavily. Snort and grunt. Use lots of lube as you jerk off. Every now and then, hold the phone right by your prick so he gets an earful of your juicy squelching hand strokes. When you cum, scream the house down.

Sometimes, you may feel inclined to meet up with a man you've contacted via a sex line or small ad. That may not be such a good idea. Because phone partners tend to exaggerate their physique and sexual prowess, the reality will rarely live up to your mental image. Is it worth your probable disappointment and the shattering of your enjoyable fantasy?

Watching and showing off

There are guys who get erotic gratification watching other men get undressed or commit sexual acts. There are those who are turned on by other men looking at them taking off their clothes or having sex.

Respectively known as 'voyeurism' and 'exhibitionism', these forms of fetish are quite harmless, providing everyone's aware what's going on and participates with free consent. Flashing and peeping at unwilling people is, of course, not consensual. Given that visual stimulation is such an important part of erotic arousal, there is an element of watching and showing off in nearly all sexual encounters.

It exists when partners get a thrill from watching each other climax, or from taking photographs of themselves in the nude. There is also a whisper of exhibitionism about kissing in a crowded place, jerking off in front of a mirror, or sex in any open air setting such as a beach or mountain top. Much of the fun of jerk off parties is based on the excitement of watching other guys cum, and being watched by them. Given the widespread consumption of porno magazines and videos, not to mention homoerotic images in mainstream advertising, most of us are voyeurs nowadays.

Piercing

Piercing is a form of eroticized body decoration. The most common piercings are studs in the tongue and lips, and rings or barbells through the nipples, cock and balls. For guys who are turned on by piercing, it stimulates arousal, highlights particularly pleasurable erogenous zones, and intensifies the enjoyment of sex. Nipple rings, for example, are often worn as a way of keeping tits erect, drawing attention to them, advertising enjoyment of tit play, and making it easier for tits to be teased and pulled.

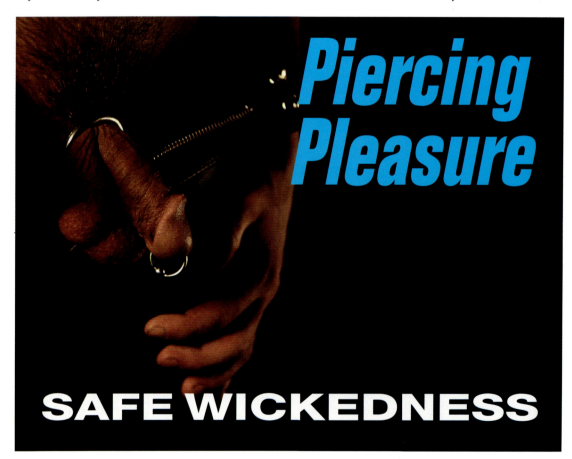

Piercing Pleasure — SAFE WICKEDNESS

Safe piercing

Never try to pierce yourself. Have it done by a registered professional using sterilized equipment and surgical steel jewellery. Non-sterile instruments can pass on HIV and hepatitis; poor quality jewellery can cause metal poisoning. If you are having sex with a pierced partner, be careful not to pull or bite his piercings too hard. This could cause splits and bleeding, which may put you both at risk of HIV. Never swap piercing jewellery unless you have first boiled and disinfected it.

Shaving

Smooth, boyish bodies can look very attractive, and feel fabulous with their all-over silky softness. For these reasons, some men like to remove body hair. A few find the act of being shaved a powerful aphrodisiac. They get off on the state of being passive and vulnerable while another man delicately fondles and grooms their body with a lethal blade. Having armpits, chest, butt, dick and balls smothered with warm foam, and experiencing a cold razor sensuously slice away body hair, can be hugely arousing.

Safe shaving

Use a new razor. Don't share it with your partner. Blood can spread infection. If you get cut, clean and cover the wound before you get down to sex.

Piss

Warm splashes of golden piss trickling down the face and chest are a big turn-on for some guys. The excitement comes from being drenched in someone else's intimate body fluids. This isn't a million miles from the thrill that most of us get from having another guy shoot his cum over our body.

Sexual activities involving piss – often called watersports or golden showers – usually take place in the bath, which makes it easy to wash off afterwards.

Pissing is something you can enjoy many more times a night than you can have orgasms. All you need to do is drink a lot! Consuming a large volume of liquid ensures your piss is fragrant, not foul.

Safe pissing

It is completely safe to have a guy piss on you, from head to toe, providing you keep your eyes closed and have no open skin wounds. However, piss can sometimes contain traces of blood. So, there is a small risk of HIV if piss gets in your mouth or eyes, and a larger risk if he pisses up your arse. Other infections can also be passed on in piss. Getting gonorrhoea in your eyes can, for example, cause blindness if it is not treated promptly.

Shit

Shitting on another guy, or being shitted on, smearing bodies with shit, or eating it – this sexual ritualization of shit is nick-named 'scat'. The medical term is 'coprophilia'.

It is often part of a humiliation scene where men get sexually aroused by suffering degradation and indignity, or by inflicting it. However, shit play can also be a form of adoration in which lust or love for another man extends to worshipping everything about him.

Our attitudes towards shit are culturally influenced. In a society which makes the arse taboo, it is hardly surprising that shit is despised. So, too, is licking and fucking arse. Yet these activities give many gay men great satisfaction, despite often involving contact with traces of excrement.

The extreme revulsion against the arse and its contents is irrational. Shitting is a natural part of life and is essential for good health. This doesn't mean we have an obligation to enjoy playing with shit, but it does mean we ought to keep our attitudes towards others who enjoy it in proper perspective.

Safe shitting

Having fun with shit is safe, if it doesn't enter the body. This means it is safe to smear it over yourself providing your skin is undamaged. But it's not safe to eat shit, get shit on open wounds, or get someone else's shit inside your arse or down your piss-hole.

Shit is very risky for hepatitis A and B, and for intestinal infections like giardiasis. It is very low risk for HIV, unless it contains blood. However, since blood in shit is not always noticeable, it's safest to avoid all shit play which could allow the virus to enter the body.

Another option is switching to shit fantasies using safe substitutes such as bratwurst, black olives, peanut butter or chocolate.

Fisting

For some guys who enjoy big dicks, having a whole fist and forearm up their arse is a logical extension to their desire for bigness. Fisting, or fist-fucking as it is often called, gives a feeling of fullness, and massages the insides, in a way that is beyond the power of even the largest cock. It's a size fantasy come true.

The thrill of fisting also derives from the element of domination and submission it involves. The person being fisted is vulnerable and at the mercy of the fister. Both partners experience, from different

Safer Sexy
Diversity and Spice

perspectives, an exhilarating sense of controlled physical power as the fist works its way deep into the arse.

Safe fisting

Fist-fucking can be quite safe, providing the person being fisted is fully relaxed and no force is used, and providing the person doing the fisting has smooth nails and no cuts on his hand or arm. However, without care, fist-fucking can tear the lining of the butt and result in very serious internal injuries.

If you want to be fist-fucked, choose a partner who has experience of being fisted himself, so he knows how to do it carefully. Don't get out of your mind on drink or drugs. Ensure you remain clear-headed and in control so your are able to avoid forced penetration and recognize any internal damage if it occurs.

If you are the guy doing the fisting:

- File your nails short and smooth.
- Remove any rings, bracelets or watches.
- Wear rubber gloves, if you have any cuts or abrasions on your hand or arm.
- Use lots of lubrication, preferably not oil-based, on both his arse and your hand.
- Get the guy being fisted to take long, deep breaths to help untense his muscles.
- Penetrate very slowly and gently, starting with one finger and then adding extra fingers as he gets more relaxed.
- Stop every now and then to allow him to get used to your inward movement.
- Once you are fully inside, your fisting motion should be a sensuous massage, not a violent thrusting action.
- Don't penetrate deeper than ten inches (twenty five centimetres), which about the maximum that any arse can safely take.

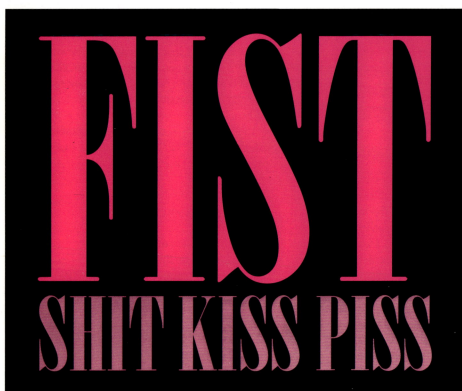

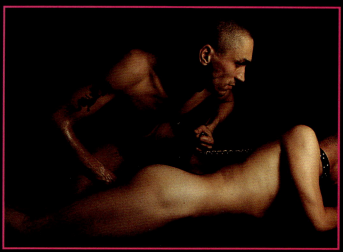

**Whatever turns you on
Enjoy it safely**

Diversity and Spice
Sadomasochism

♂ If he feels pain, or you notice blood, stop immediately and very slowly withdraw your hand. If pain or blood persist, seek urgent medical attention.

♂ Once you have finished fisting, wash your hand and arm before touching anything else (to clean off any traces of blood or shit).

♂ If you have used oil-based lube for fisting, don't fuck afterwards; the oil may cause the condom to break.

Sadomasochism

Sadomasochism (S and M, or SM) is more about power than pain. It's the achievement of mutual pleasure from freely consenting behaviour involving domination and submission, where one partner exercizes control over another. The dominant guy gets a surge of lust or a mental buzz from wielding power. His submissive partner is sexually aroused or psychologically fulfilled by being powerless, vulnerable and dependent.

SM encompasses a wide spectrum of activities embodying various degrees of domination, including punishment, bondage, degradation and, in extreme cases, serious pain. Not all of these are overtly sexual. Some, like flogging, may not involve genital contact nor lead to orgasm. What they all have in common is the stimulation of shared erotic or emotional enjoyment through opposite, but complementary, desires to conquer and surrender.

Although pain can be a part of SM, often the acts of domination and submission revolve around painless sex play based on physical restraint and confinement, such as being tied up or caged, and around psychological humiliation like boot-licking, verbal abuse and shit scenes.

When SM does include elements of pain, it is

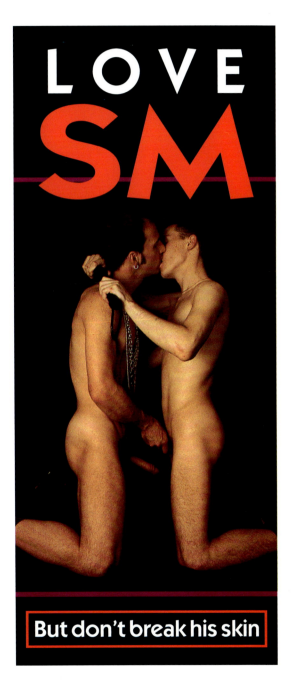

LOVE SM
But don't break his skin

mostly limited to the mild levels of tit biting, arse spanking and ball squeezing. The infliction of severe pain, as with violent whipping and genital mutilation, is less common.

In other words, SM primarily concerns the ritualization and eroticization of power within a relationship. This is done through the acting out of strongly contrasting sex roles. The dominant partner is known as the top or master. He gets his kicks from leading and controlling the action and from performing any sexual penetration involved. The submissive partner is called the bottom or slave. He's the guy who enjoys being led and controlled, and who is penetrated if fucking with dildoes, fists or dicks is part of the action.

The act of domination doesn't always have connotations of violation, roughness and discomfort. Sometimes, the domination may be of a more playful teasing nature, with a good deal of ribbing and tantalizing but no physical aggression. On other occasions, it can be domination of a protective, gentle and soothing nature. The submissive partner is lovingly overwhelmed with passion and pampering, as in baby-nappy-nursery fantasies.

In its purest form, the act of submission is one of martyr-like self-sacrifice. A guy gives his body to another man. He renounces his own desires for the sake of his partner's. Submission can, however, also be more pro-active and even manipulative. A slave may be demanding to the point where his master is constantly working overtime to fulfil his need to be dominated. In such circumstances, who is dominating who?

SM roles are usually confined to sex, and don't reflect how the participants behave in everyday life. Most slaves only serve their masters sexually. In other aspects of their lives, they treat each other as equals.

SM is very different from genuinely coercive and exploitative acts. The latter take place without mutual consent. The victim has no control over what

Diversity and Spice — Safer Sexy

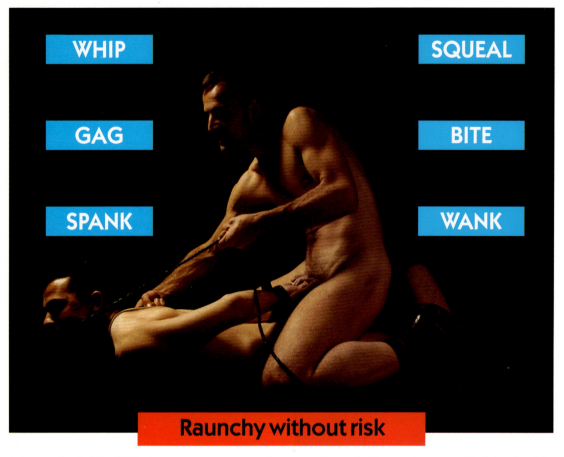

Raunchy without risk

is happening to him. SM is, in contrast, a consensual relationship between partners where one consciously chooses to submit to the will of another and be controlled by them. The guy being dominated retains the ultimate control of being able to stop the action at any time by using the safeword. This is the pre-arranged signal that either partner can use during the action to indicate that he has reached his limit and wants to stop.

At the level of cultural meaning, SM is the transgression of 'normal' desires, and the exploration of forbidden feelings. SM allows us to get in touch with sensations which are not supposed to be enjoyable, but which can be. SM is sexually subversive. Nasty is nice, and vice versa.

Breaking down the mental barriers we erect to police our libido, SM brings to life deep, repressed sexual longings. In place of our carefully controlled selves, it allows us to lose control within a safe context. The artificial, contrived facade of a public persona is stripped away to reveal a genuine inner self, unencumbered by the forced sexual manners of polite society.

SM can also be the managed expression of potentially dangerous and threatening fantasies. Rules and safewords set limits to keep it safe. This can give people the confidence to explore feelings they may otherwise be afraid of confronting. A guy who wants to be sexually ravaged while bound and gagged may be more willing to put himself in that situation of vulnerability if he knows his submission is for a limited duration – and can be stopped whenever he has had enough.

Maybe more people should explore SM. By acknowledging and acting out desires of domination, discomfort and degradation in controlled and safe ways, it is arguable that SM could, for some men, provide a safety valve to prevent those desires exploding in uncontrolled and dangerous ways which might cause genuine damage and suffering. The process of ritualizing sexual domination and violence can provide an outlet which diffuses its menace. Someone with recurrent fantasies either of raping or being raped, for example, may find that an SM scenario involving simulated rape could help manage those desires in a way that is mutually fulfilling, instead of being harmful.

Furthermore, the accentuated role-playing of SM encounters can provide relief from the pressures of real-life situations. A senior government official might long for release from the burdens and responsibilities of his demanding job. As the subordinate partner in an SM relationship, he may get much relief and satisfaction from letting someone else take charge and thereby absolving himself of all responsibilities.

SM involves great honesty. Partners open up to each other about desires that most people keep hidden. But it requires a huge amount of trust. Putting oneself in a vulnerable situation, where harm is possible if things get out of hand, is a demonstration of immense confidence in another person. A slave being humiliated is totally dependent on his master knowing how far to go and when to stop.

Diversity and Spice
Sadomasochism

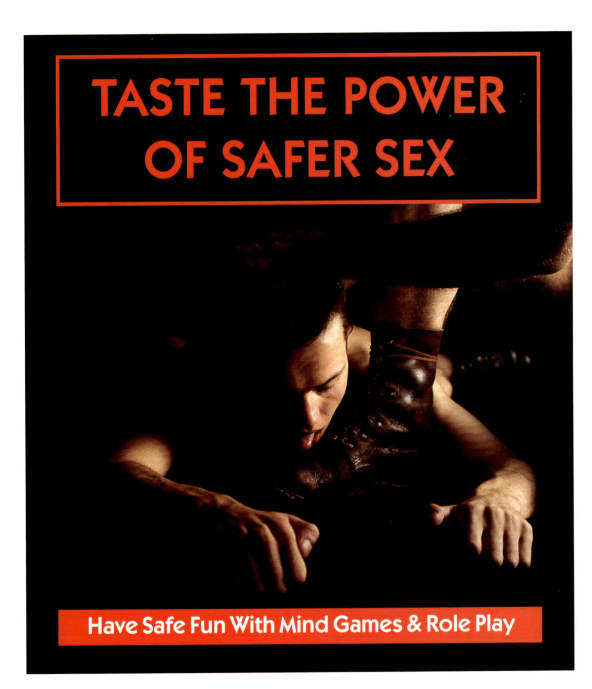

In lots of ways the difference between SM and non-SM is not as clear cut as many people think. All relationships involve elements of domination and submission. What SM does is to honestly acknowledge, and then exalt, ritualize and exaggerate this everyday power-play between partners.

Most of us incorporate aspects of SM into our sex lives; whether it be a bit of tit squeezing, or occasional physical restraint. This begs the question: how hard and how often do you have to squeeze a guy's tits or constrain his body before it qualifies as SM? This crossover and ambiguity is also evident in fashion where the SM imagery of metal-studded belts and leather jeans has become commonplace style, although SM fashion doesn't necessarily indicate SM practice. In the bedroom, SM paraphernalia such as handcuffs and harnesses are now a part of many people's sexual routines.

Safe SM

Most SM is very safe from the point of view of HIV and other sexually-transmitted diseases. The only risk is from SM acts that penetrate the body, draw blood or serum, and play with body fluids. These include activities like fisting, caning and pissing. Before starting a SM session, always agree to stick to safer sex and prevent the exchange of blood, serum and cum.

The other safety guidelines are that SM should always be undertaken with informed consent, without causing permanent harm, and with a predetermined safeword so the action can be halted if it gets too strong. Avoid safewords like 'Stop!'. If you are being whipped, begging your master to stop may be part of your role. Choose an unobvious safeword, like your own name. Then he will know for sure when you have had enough.

When you first try SM, it is very important to choose an experienced and trusted partner, ideally someone known and recommended by a friend.

Safer Sexy
Diversity and spice

Finally, SM doesn't mix with drugs and alcohol. Being out of your head can make you careless. This is extremely dangerous when you are doing things involving pain and bondage, where the safety of the other person is dependent on your good judgement. If you or your partner are high, save the pleasures of SM for another time.

Bondage

What is the difference between your partner fucking you while holding your hands behind your head, and fucking you while your hands are tied to the bed? It's a matter of degrees.

Tying up a sexual partner with ropes and handcuffs, or restraining his physical movement in other ways using mouth gags, slings, ankle straps, racks, chains, strait-jackets, hoods, and cages, is the most extreme form of erotic domination. One partner is totally at the mercy of another, which is why some men find it so arousing. The real thrill of bondage comes from the tension between power, dependence, violation and trust.

The guy who agrees to be constrained hands over control. He entrusts another man with the care of his body and the satisfaction of his desires. However, like other forms of SM, both guys agree on a pre-arranged signal, the safeword, to stop the action when the guy tied up has had enough. The man who ties up his partner and assumes absolute control over him, gets his sexual rush from being able to do whatever he wants – bite, fuck, kiss, slap, jerk or anything else that takes his fancy, subject to limits imposed by safer sex and the safeword. For the guy who is tied up, this uncertainty about what might be done to him adds to the sexual intoxication.

The sensation of being bound can be very caring, protective and comforting. Some men describe it as being like a warm constricting embrace, not dissimilar to being squeezed very tight by someone you love. At the other extreme, bondage can be a violent imprisoning humiliation. It all depends on what turns you on, and how you and your partner decide to play the game. Whichever way you experience it, having an orgasm while in a state of helplessness, where all you can do is groan and writhe, is very different from cumming without any physical restraint.

Bondage also has a social symbolism. It's the conscious disavowal of sexual free will. A guy who is physically immobilized is powerless. He has no control over the sexual action, having surrendered all decision-making and responsibility to his partner. In making explicit the absence of sexual free will, bondage merely accentuates an aspect of all carnal relations. When do we ever have unrestricted erotic choice? Is not the scope of our sexual freedom always shaped and limited by long forgotten past experiences, and by never recognized unconscious desires? Bondage is merely the honest representation, in heightened and ritualized form, of these restraints on our capacity for sexual free will.

Safe bondage

Being tied up is in itself no-risk for HIV and other sexual infections. But unsafe sexual acts during bondage are dangerous. It's very important to agree before you begin a bondage scene that any fucking will be with a condom. Other safe bondage tips include:

⚭ While bound and gagged, you are vulnerable to being robbed or bashed. Never let yourself be tied up by someone unless you have first introduced him to a friend, and preferably not until you know him well enough to be certain you trust him. Whenever you meet up with a guy for bondage fun, leave his name, address and phone number with a friend, and discreetly let him know that is what you have done.

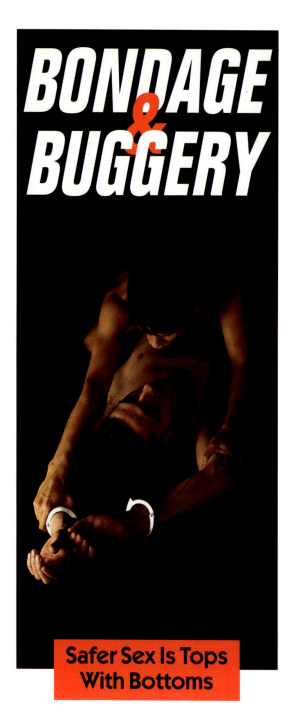

BONDAGE & BUGGERY

Safer Sex Is Tops With Bottoms

Diversity and Spice
Pain pleasure

Pain pleasure

In a lot of sex there is an interplay between pleasure and pain. The experience of one helps define and accentuate the experience of the other. Overcoming the initial pain of being fucked, for example, produces incredible relief which magnifies the subsequent pleasure. To some extent, therefore, it is through the knowledge of pain that the joy of pleasure is maximized and appreciated.

However, there are also moments when the contrast between pleasure and pain becomes blurred. Arse-slapping, love-bites and nipple-pinching all involve elements of mild pain which most guys find erotically enjoyable.

Some SM enthusiasts develop this pain pleasure into more intense forms, such as whipping and puncturing. These types of SM explore the boundaries of pain and pleasure and the limits of personal endurance. Skilled pain pleasure involves the random mixing of pain and pleasure to create sexual tension and excitement. Soft, sensual caresses are suddenly replaced by a stinging cat o' nine tails. This unexpected switch from comforting, reassuring gentleness to shocking, violating pain can produce an exhilarating, unnerving adrenaline rush and sexual high. It's not unlike the thrill of a roller coaster ride where the tension between the long calmness of slowly climbing upwards and the sudden terror of rapidly plunging downwards is the key to the enjoy-

- Strangulation and suffocation activities are risky. Too often they end in tragedy. Don't tie anything around the neck. Use your hands. Never let your partner lose consciousness. In case things go wrong, learn how to give effective mouth-to-mouth resuscitation.

- It's best not to suspend guys from their wrists or ankles for long periods as this may harm circulation. Even shortterm suspensions should only be undertaken if you have padded constraints to protect against compression damage to the nerves and tendons.

- Be very careful with face hoods, masks and gags. Ensure the person wearing them is able to breathe, and can indicate if he wants you to stop. If restraints prevent him from saying the safeword, prearrange an alternative signal such as three grunts or three nods of the head. Always stop when he says so.

- Don't tie knots too tight, or keep a guy tied up for too long. During lengthy bondage, change the restraints every now and then. Otherwise you might stop circulation, damage nerves, and cause muscle and joint aches.

- Look out for differences in skin colour either side of a restraint. If tied up body parts go dark, or feel cold, it's a sign that the restraints are cutting off the blood supply. Loosen them immediately.

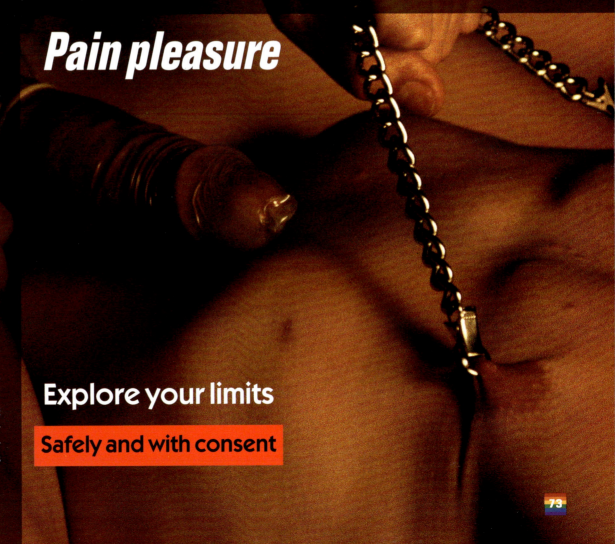

Pain pleasure

Explore your limits

Safely and with consent

Diversity and Spice — Safer Sexy

GET WISE & PRICK PROUD

ment. These same elements of tension, uncertainty and sharply contrasting sensations are central to some guys' pleasure in hurtful SM.

There are graduations of pleasurable pain. Spanking is one of the mildest and simplest. All it takes is an open palm and a good whack on the arse, as soft or as hard as your partner prefers. Canes and whips offer sweet agony several degrees stronger. Spanking and other forms of beating are rarely just physical acts. Usually they are part of a domination-submission mind game, such as corporal punishment where a 'naughty schoolboy' or 'AWOL sailor' is ritually chastised.

Most pain-inducing SM is limited to the mild to moderate levels of tit-clamps and hot candle wax. Only rarely does it extend to extreme forms of genital torture. Be mindful that in Britain and some other countries even consensual SM is illegal if it involves physical injury.

Safe pain pleasure

Painful activities that don't penetrate your body or break the skin are safe from HIV. But there are other dangers to avoid:

⚭ Before you start any pain-inflicting SM session, agree a signal (safeword) to stop when you or your partner have had enough, and agree to limit the action to superficial wounds which do not cause any longterm injury or scars.

⚭ If you are into flogging, aim your blows at fleshy areas of the body like the arse and thighs to prevent damage to bones, tendons, nerves and internal organs. Watch for cuts and bruises, and avoid repeatedly flogging any area that shows signs of injury.

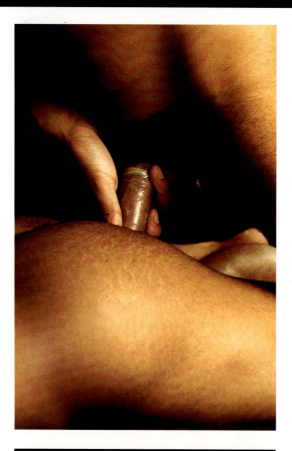

When You Pull Out Hold Tight To The Rubber

⚭ Beatings with whips or canes may cut the skin and cause bleeding or release serum (a clear liquid that can also carry HIV). Never share whips or canes. Always use a new one each time, or thoroughly wash and disinfect it between partners even if there are no visible signs of blood or serum.

⚭ Puncturing, abrading or burning the skin can be dangerous. It creates wounds which may get infected, and can leave permanent scars. Wounds spread blood, which can spread HIV. Disinfect and cover any broken skin to protect you both.

⚭ Sterilize all torture implements before use and never swop them with your partner.

⚭ As well as the danger of infection, puncturing the body with things like needles and nails could injure nerve endings and cause disfigurement. To avoid the dangers of do-it-yourself piercing, get your body parts pierced by a qualified professional.

⚭ If you like hanging weights from your tits, cock or balls, be careful not to overdo it. Otherwise, you could end up with perpetually sagging flesh.

⚭ Don't cum over any body-part where skin is damaged. If you shoot cum over a guy after a flogging or puncturing session, be careful your spunk doesn't trickle down into the area of broken skin when he moves about after sex.

⚭ Remember, there is a safe way to do every type of sexual activity. With a little imagination and common sense you can enjoy the most ordinary and the most unusual erotic acts endlessly, and risk-free.

Sex Problems and Solutions
Inability to cum

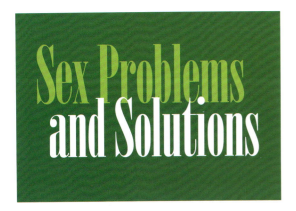

Sex Problems and Solutions

It is quite normal for our sexual performance to vary. Most of us experience sexual problems every now and then. They are usually fleeting and quickly disappear of their own accord. We soon get over them.

Sometimes, however, sexual difficulties persist, which can play havoc with relationships. The good news is that nearly all these difficulties are resolvable, as long as they are faced up to and the necessary remedial action is taken.

The majority of sexual problems are psychological, not physical. They usually respond well to self-help exercises, although some may need the help of a professional sex therapist.

Cumming too fast

Referred to by doctors as 'premature ejaculation', cumming too fast involves reaching sexual climax sooner than desired, and often without experiencing a full-strength orgasm. It's caused by an inability to control physical responses to sexual excitement. With practice these responses are controllable.

There are four techniques which can help solve the problem of cumming too quick. They can be used individually or in combination.

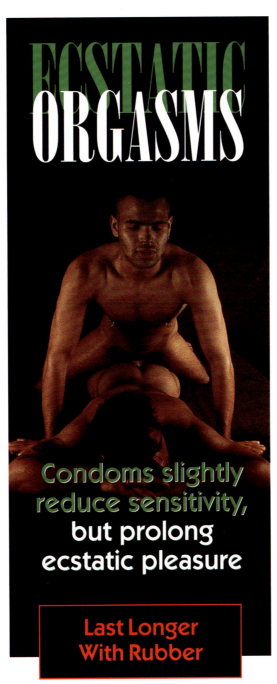

Condoms slightly reduce sensitivity, but prolong ecstatic pleasure

Last Longer With Rubber

Sensitivity reduction

Orgasm can be delayed by reducing the sensitivity of your cock. This can be achieved by wearing an extra thick condom and using an anaesthetizing cream. Jerking off every day, and shortly before you meet a guy for sex, will also lower the build up of sexual energy and slightly dull erotic excitation. Although useful, these three ways to reduce sensitivity are superficial solutions which do not solve the underlying problem of uncontrollable over-quick reactions to sexual stimulation.

Mental distraction

Cumming too fast is partly psychological; the brain receives erotic sensations from the dick and sends signals back which trigger involuntary rapid orgasm. Focusing your mind on something non-sexual, like working out the ingredients needed for tomorrow night's dinner, is a way of interrupting the signals between the brain and the cock which set off a premature climax. It effectively slows down the tempo of psychological and physical arousal, which delays the orgasmic release.

Stop – start

The length of time it takes to reach orgasm is mostly a conditioned reflex. It's something we learn through experience. If a guy has a long history of hurried jerking off to avoid discovery or to please an impatient partner, it can set in motion a permanent and involuntary cycle of quick cumming. The most effective way to solve premature ejaculation is to unlearn this rapid reflex. This can be done through a series of exercises which help control the process of cumming. The stop-start method involves stopping sex just before orgasm, and then restarting it once the urge to cum has subsided. By repeating this exercise over and over, the length of time between pauses will gradually get longer. Begin this method by jerking off alone, without lubricant. Keep stop-starting for twenty minutes before letting yourself cum. Once you have achieved this goal, add lubrication to increase the level of sensitivity, and repeat the process. When you can keep this up for twenty minutes, try the same technique with an understanding and supportive partner. Choose a moment when you both have plenty of time with no pressure to rush things. Begin the stop-start exercizes with him jerking you off, and later move on to body rubbing, sucking and fucking.

Squeeze

This is a variant of the stop-start method. Whatever way you decide to have sex, when you are nearly about to cum, instead of stopping sexual activity, grasp the head of your dick and squeeze it hard. Press your thumb very tightly against the underside just below the head. Hold it for several seconds until the cumming sensation disappears and your cock loses a bit of its erection. Repeat this exercise six times before cumming. Squeezing is particularly useful if you have a lot of difficulty stopping yourself from cumming when you use the stop-start method.

Whichever of these techniques or combinations of techniques you use, don't expect major changes overnight. It will take weeks, and possibly months. Nevertheless, it's worth the persistence – you'll end up with a more fulfiling sex life.

Inability to cum

An inability to cum, or excessive slowness in reaching orgasm, is known medically as 'retarded ejaculation'. Most guys with this condition have no difficulty climaxing when they jerk off alone. It is only with a partner they have problems. Sometimes it's not a total inability to cum. They may be able to climax when being jerked or sucked, but not when fucking.

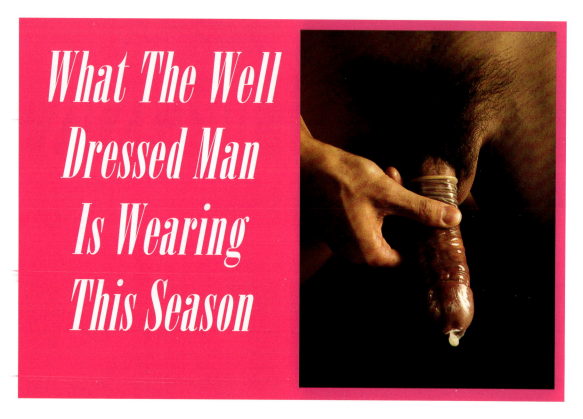

What The Well Dressed Man Is Wearing This Season

The cause is muscular over-control. Usually this has psychological origins such as stress, tiredness, sexual guilt, performance anxiety or bad feelings between partners. These influences involuntarily generate brain waves that unconsciously block the muscular reactions which are necessary for sexual climax. Once a pattern of prolonged inability to reach orgasm is established, you need to retrain your cumming reflex to overcome the problem. This involves a series of desensitizing exercises which gradually reduce your sensitivity to the things that inhibit your climax. You start with sex in a situation that causes you no worry and does not impair your sexual ability. Then, step-by-step, you progress to sex in circumstances that would normally provoke anxiety and prevent you from cumming. By repeating these exercises over and over, most guys can eventually conquer slowness in reaching orgasm. If you have no problem cumming when you jerk off yourself alone, but find it hard to climax with another guy, try the stage-by-stage desensitization method. Make sure your partner is someone you trust and feel comfortable with. It's very important to do the following exercises with a guy who understands your difficulties and will take the time necessary to help you remedy them. As you successfully accomplish one stage, move on to the next.

Sex Problems and Solutions
Lack of erection

Step-by-step exercises

♂ Start with you and your partner jerking off simultaneously in separate rooms – first with the doors closed, and later with them open so you can hear each other's groans and panting.

♂ Jerk off yourselves in opposite corners of the same room, facing away from each other.

♂ Each time you succeed in cumming, move a little closer to your partner until you are back to back.

♂ Turn to reposition yourselves side by side as you jerk off, and then face to face.

♂ Caress and kiss one another while jerking off, but do not touch each other's dicks.

♂ Jerk yourself off until your climax is just past the point of no return and then get your partner to finish you off, either by jerking or sucking.

♂ Gradually let him take over at an ever earlier stage in your sexual arousal.

♂ Once you are able to cum with him sucking and jerking you, progress to fucking your partner as you near orgasm (put a condom on your dick soon after you get hard – this avoids interrupting the flow of the action).

Lack of erection

Failure to get or maintain an erection, known medically as 'impotence', is something all of us experience from time to time. It can result from a lack of sexual attraction or compatibility, excess alcohol, drug use, sickness, medication, tension, guilt about sex or being gay, relationship problems, bereavement, nervousness with a new partner, the stress of unemployment, or the physical malfunction of our arousal process.

There are also periods when sex loses its attraction. Our interest wanes. Perhaps we are preoccupied with an exciting creative or business venture or some other all-consuming project. Maybe we have a physically weak sex drive or have been through a period of erotic saturation and over-indulgence. Whatever the reason, it's okay to feel non-sexual.

Occasional erection difficulties are nothing to worry about. We all have our ups and downs. If your partner isn't able to get aroused, be understanding and supportive. You can still give him the pleasure of lots of kisses and caresses. Avoid pressurising him to perform. That will only make things worse.

When a guy repeatedly fails to get a hard-on and feels under pressure from his partner, it can create an escalating spiral of increased anxiety which further diminishes his capacity for stiffness. Every successive failure makes him more anxious to perform and therefore less likely to succeed.

A man's inability to get an erection, especially with guys he would normally fancy, is usually due to mental barriers. To resolve psychologically-rooted erection loss, it's vital to find ways of learning not to worry. Worry exacerbates the problem. If you have hard on difficulties, the following desensitising exercises will help you relax and remove any pressure to perform.

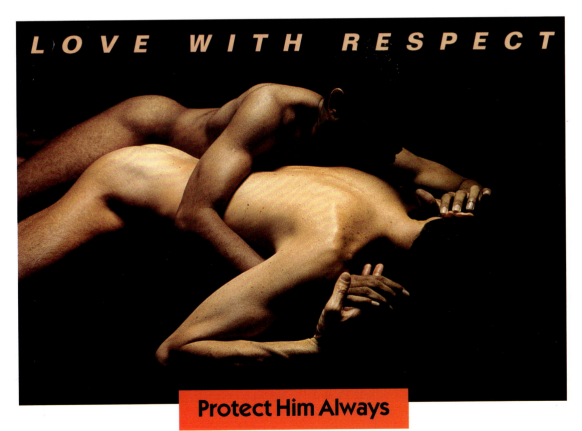

Safer Sexy
Sex Problems and Solutions

Step-by-step exercises

☙ Abstain from sex, including jerking off, for two weeks.

☙ Then choose a caring, patient partner. Agree with him that whatever happens during these exercises you will not have sex.

☙ Get him to start by sensually massaging your whole body without touching your cock. Forget about getting hard and cumming. Relax. Concentrate on enjoying the erotic sensations.

☙ Next, have your partner massage your dick and balls. Whenever you become stiff, get him to stop until you go limp again. Then have him resume the massage. By repeating this process of gaining and losing an erection over and over, your anxiety about erection loss will gradually fade.

☙ Finally, when you have repeated these exercises many times and begun to go hard spontaneously, at the end of the each session let your partner bring you to orgasm.

In addition to psychological causes, the inability to get an erection sometimes has physical origins, such as damage to the nerve connections which send signals back and forth between the brain and cock, or obstructions to the blood flow which is needed for the dick to swell.

There are three possible solutions to the problem of physical impotence. First, using micro-surgery, faulty nerves and blood arteries can sometimes be repaired. Second, just before sex, a drug can be injected into the dick, which will trigger a hard-on lasting up to several hours. Third, semi-hard rods can be surgically implanted into the cavity chambers of the cock to create a permanent stiffness. These rods can be rigid or flexible. The bendy type allows the prick to be bent outwards during sex and bent downwards for pissing. Another implant method involves inflatable cylinders being inserted in the dick. These are connected to a fluid reservoir implanted in the abdomen and a tiny pump implanted in the ball sac. Squeezing the pump forces liquid into the cock, producing an erection. When sex is over, a switch on the pump is used to return the fluid to the reservoir, thereby deflating the dick.

Sex compulsion

Sexual desire is healthy. Sexual compulsion is not. What constitutes a healthy amount of sex varies from one person to the next. Some guys have a stronger sex drive than others, or more opportunities and better luck. There are those for whom jerking off twice a day and picking up men four times a week is normal. For others, it may seem excessive.

There is nothing wrong with having lots of sex. It's only a problem if it gets out of control and disrupts a person's life. Sexual compulsion is when sex ceases to be one of several enjoyable aspects of life and becomes a totally dominating and uncontrollable obsession which is never satisfied no matter how many partners and how good the orgasms. When a guy is addicted to sex, he has to have it constantly regardless of the place, time or consequences.

This incessant quest for sexual partners twenty four hours a day interferes with work, relationships and social life. It may cause financial hardship as income is swallowed up on bar-hopping, saunas, contact ads, sex phone lines, and porno magazines and videos.

When sex completely dominates a man's life, he needs to ask why. What inner longing, or loathing, is causing such irrational and self-destructive behaviour? Is it a fear of falling in love and then suffering the emotional hurt of breaking up? Is it compensation for an aimless life or a lack of love? Is it an

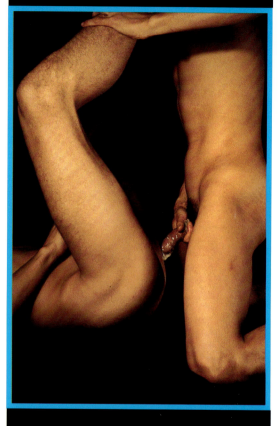

expression of low self-esteem and worthlessness? Is it anxiety that a relationship will mean a loss of independence? Is it sexual vanity and egoism?

If you feel you have a sexual compulsion that is out of control and is causing you distress, try dealing with it in the following ways:

⚣ Think about when and why you first became addicted to sex.

⚣ Concentrate on improving the quality, rather than the quantity, of your sexual encounters.

⚣ Visualize what would have to happen for you to reduce your sexual obsessiveness. What other interests could you cultivate?

⚣ Spend time developing non-sexual interests and friendships.

⚣ Seek the advice of a professional sex counsellor who can help you recognize and overcome the underlying cause of your compulsion.

Drug or alcohol dependence

Something is seriously wrong if you can't cruise and chat up guys without being high on alcohol or drugs. When you need to be off your face to get an erection and enjoy sex, it's time to stop and fathom out the reasons. Dependence on chemical buzzes often indicates lack of confidence, shame about being gay, fear of rejection and absence of self-worth. Far from solving problems, too much booze and narcotics only adds to them. It can create difficulties at work and in relationships, damage your brain and immune system, and increase the likelihood of illness, accidents and suicide.

There is, of course, a world of difference between dependence and selective use. Alcohol and most non-addictive drugs are fine when they are consumed every now and then to enhance enjoyment. However, they are not alright when they reduce a person to an incoherent, vegetative state, or when they become a substitute for an enjoyable life and a way of blotting out loneliness and depression.

On the plus side, occasional and moderate use of stimulants can variously lower inhibitions, increase sociability, or heighten sensations and energy levels. This can make nightclubs, dinner parties, sex and relationships more relaxed, adventurous and pleasurable.

However, chemical highs can sometimes have the opposite effect, making users feel anxious, withdrawn and unable to get hard-ons. A lack of sexual interest or ability is a common reaction to certain drugs and large amounts of alcohol.

Not all drugs are the same; some are safer than others. Mind-altering psychedelics like LSD can distort consciousness, which may lead to careless, risky behaviour. Addictive narcotics, such as heroin and crack, are never safe and should be totally avoided. Others are best used with care and moderation to prevent psychological dependence.

Being out of your head on alcohol or drugs impairs perception and judgement. You could pick up men

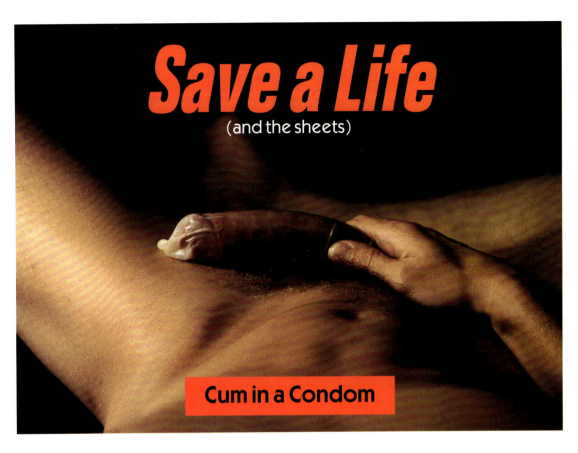

you later regret having slept with, and you are certainly more likely to have unsafe sex. Booze and narcotics make it easier to let yourself go and this can be fun, but it may result in you taking risks that you would not take if you were clear-headed.

The dangers are greatest for guys who constantly use drugs or alcohol and become dependent on them. When you cannot have a good time without a chemically-induced high, something's wrong in your life. If getting by without alcohol or drugs ceases to be an option, you're no longer in control. Your use is a compulsion, not a choice.

Check yourself for signs of dependence. Do you need drugs or alcohol to function? Has alcohol or drug use caused sexual impotence, difficulties at work or the break-up of a relationship? Is a large part of your disposable income spent on drugs or alcohol? Are you in debt because of your chemical dependence? Do you use alcohol or drugs as a way of blocking out problems and worries? If the answer to any of these questions is 'yes', you need to seek professional advice.

Safe drug use

All drugs are potentially dangerous. Even 'soft' narcotics like marijuana can, with excessive use, sometimes become psychologically addictive. If you are not certain whether you can cope with drugs, and keep their use under control, think twice before starting to use them. If you do use drugs the risks can be reduced by the following precautions:

⚭ Sharing needles and syringes can spread HIV, syphilis and hepatitis. If you inject drugs, get your own syringe and needle set. Keep it to yourself and never share it with others. Always wash and disinfect the skin before injecting. Afterwards, clean your injection set with bleach or surgical spirit, and rinse it several times with clean water. Then place it in a clean sealed container until you next use it.

⚭ Impure drugs can make you sick, and even kill you. Never buy drugs from an unknown person. Always score from a dealer you know, or a dealer recommended by a friend you trust.

⚭ Some people have very bad reactions to drugs that others tolerate easily. When you try a new drug for the first time, choose a safe environment with friends who can be relied upon to look after you should things go wrong.

⚭ If you are into body-building, don't use steroids to help put on muscle. Large doses have been linked to liver cancer, high blood pressure, reduced sex drive and sudden fits of aggression.

⚭ Stay in control and avoid dependence. Use drugs as a special treat, and not as an everyday routine (which dulls the effect). That way, you'll have something special to look forward to on your treat days, and you will get a better high and more enjoyment.

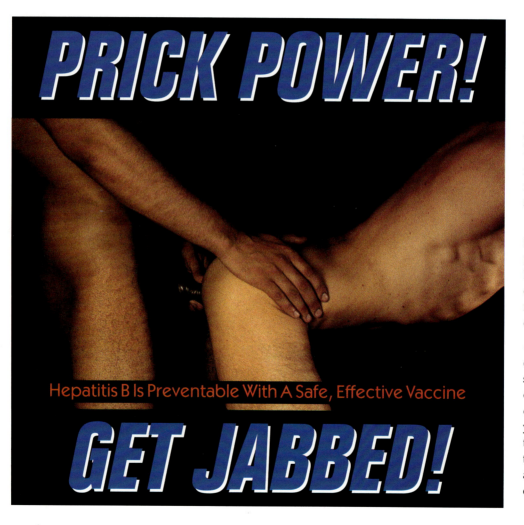

PRICK POWER! GET JABBED!
Hepatitis B Is Preventable With A Safe, Effective Vaccine

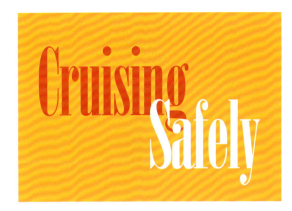

Cruising Safely

Finders, keepers. If we never seek, we never find. Sitting at home alone is no way to get a prick up your arse! And you won't find love either. The solution: cruising.

Cruising is going out to look for a man to have sex with, and possibly to fall in love with. The most obvious places to cruise are: gay venues like bars, any street or supermarket in a gay neighbourhood, and public places which are known gay rendezvous, such as certain squares, toilets, parks, railway stations, department stores, forests and beaches.

However, since gay and bisexual men are everywhere, and since some supposedly straight men are curious, cruising is something you can do any place, any time – on a train, in a shopping centre, or at a cinema.

Whenever you see a man you want to bed, don't waste time trying to work out whether he is gay or not. Who cares? Lots of queers are straight-acting and plenty of so-called straight men are open to queer sex. Unless a guy has a belligerent demeanour or is with a group of tough-looking mates, it is usually safe to cruise anyone. You will sometimes be surprised by who is available – all you have to do is approach them in the right way.

Making contact

Successful cruising is based on eye contact and smiles; plus a friendly, relaxed and confident attitude. Guys who come across as tense, awkward or desperate usually go home alone. Trying to trick is a gamble. Sometimes you win, sometimes you lose. You have the right to ask, he has the right to refuse (and vice versa). Most times, the worst that can happen is being turned down. Even then, you may get a buzz from having at least tried. Don't get too upset. There's always another cruiseable guy just round the next corner.

The techniques for cruising outdoors in the street and indoors in a gay venue are basically the same, but with slight variations.

Cruising the streets

When you are walking and you see a guy you fancy coming your way, lock your eyes on him with a friendly deliberate stare. But don't stop. Keep walking. After you've passed each other, look back at him. If he has ignored you, keep walking and forget him. But if he glances back at you, especially more than once, he may be interested. To find out, return his glances with a smile. This helps relax him. It signals your friendly intentions; it reassures him you're

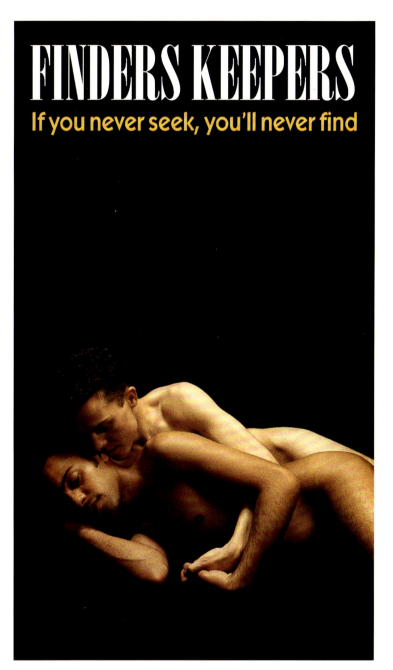

FINDERS KEEPERS
If you never seek, you'll never find

Cruising Safely — **Safer Sexy**

PICK UP HUNKS

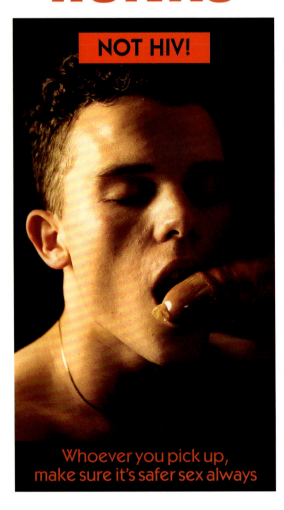

NOT HIV!

Whoever you pick up, make sure it's safer sex always

not a gay-basher. It also signifies that you are interested and approachable. He'll probably smile at you.

Should you continue to get positive feedback from the man you are cruising, stop to look in a shop window. If he stops too, keep up the eye contacts and smiles. When you get them reciprocated several times, it means he wants to get to know you.

Go over and talk to him. What you say can be about anything. Ask him if he shops in the store or comment on the merchandise in the shop window. Alternatively, seek directions to the main street or to the nearest public telephone. Or, just be bold and say hello. Then, when you have broken the ice, invite him to join you for a stroll or a drink.

Once you have seen him close up and spent a while speaking to him, you might change your mind. Perhaps you sense there is something dangerous about him. Maybe you don't fancy him after all. No problem. All you need is a plausible excuse and a polite exit line, such as: 'I have to finish some work at home. I need to get going. It was nice meeting you'.

Cruising the bars

In a gay bar or club, it is crucial to position yourself in a place where you can easily make eye contact; so that you're able to see other guys and they are able to see you. When you spy a delicious man, look straight at him to let him know you're interested. Avoid cold, unfriendly stares. Start with some warm, admiring visual seduction. Look directly into his eyes with a lingering enticing glance, and then look away. Repeat this a few times. If he returns your attention by making eye contact, it may be a sign of mutual attraction. It's worth exploring some more.

Move to within about three metres of him. This is a safe and accessible distance from which you can continue to cruise him without being intimidatingly close. It gives you both a better chance to size each other up, and to confirm or cancel your initial interest. Watch how he reacts to you moving closer. If he continues to eye you over, give him a smile. If he responds by smiling too, it usually means that he's open to being approached. Wander over and talk to him. For an opening line you could simply ask his name or tell him yours. Other options are to compliment him on his clothes, or to comment on the decor or music of the venue.

Checking him over

The process of checking out the guy you're chatting up, to make sure you are both interested in each other, is much the same wherever you happen to be cruising.

If the man you've just met is talkative, smiles a lot, and maintains eye contact, it's a very encouraging sign. A swelling in his crotch is a bonus. Move very close to him, so your bodies are touching slightly. As the conversation progresses, occasionally rest your hand on his arm or shoulder. Discreetly and gently press against him. Be careful not to be overpowering. Should he reciprocate your intimate behaviour, it nearly always means there is shared sexual chemistry. At this point, you can tell him you fancy him and start talking about sex. Be a little oblique at first, until you are sure he is comfortable with explicit talk.

When the situation is reversed, and you are being cruised by a guy you want, it is very important to positively reinforce his overtures. Otherwise, he may assume you are not interested and move on to someone else. Return his eye contact and smiles. If he moves closer, you do the same. When he touches your body, touch him back. Don't leave him to do all the talking. Initiate conversation yourself. Ask him questions. Offer to buy him a drink. Let him know you like him.

If you are being heavily cruised by someone you're not interested in, there are a number of get-

Cruising Safely
Coping with rejection

away options. If he has not already begun conversation with you, it's easier. Just move elsewhere, or make smalltalk with another guy to put him off. If he has been chatting you up for a while, politely thank him for his flattering interest and make your exit: 'Thanks for the chat. It's been enjoyable. I'm going to take a wander now. Have a good evening!'

Sometimes, of course, the boot is on the other foot. You are cruising a man who's not interested in you, or who's changed his mind. Watch out for the warning signs. These include avoidance of eye contact, absence of smiles, one-word replies to your questions, failure to initiate conversation, resistance to physical touch, moving away from you when you move close to him, and roving eyes that wander over every guy who comes into view. If you get these signals, persist for a while to make sure he's not just shy or nervous. But when they continue with no obvious indications of interest, forget it. Things are not going to work out. Time to move on to someone who'll appreciate you.

An unfriendly and uncommunicative attitude, together with an absence of reciprocated touch, may occasionally indicate something more sinister than sexual disinterest. Or, maybe he's friendly but you sense he isn't sincere. These can be danger signals that you are cruising a straight thug who is posing as gay in order to get picked up so he can blackmail, attack or rob you.

To avoid this risk it is a sensible idea to spend a while talking with a guy before you go home together. It is also a good way to get yourselves feeling relaxed and at ease with each other. You can make sure he's into safer sex and that you are both sexually compatible. Sex is not much fun if one of you has a special sexual fetish that the other doesn't enjoy. Be sure he is giving you friendly, safe vibes. If there's any doubt, make your exit. You don't want to end up a victim of violence.

Coping with rejection

Cruising is like your dick. It has its ups and downs. Sometimes you succeed, sometimes you don't. However, if you never try, you'll never score. If everyone waited for other guys to approach them, no one would ever pick up. The more you cruise, the more experienced and skilled you become and the more likely you are to succeed. Guys who get rejected but carry on cruising have a higher success rate than those who give up after the first couple of failed attempts. It stands to reason that if you cruise five men in a night you will have a much better chance of scoring than if you only cruise only one, or none.

Even in a worst case scenario, it is often better to chat up five guys and get rejected by all of them than to spend the whole evening by yourself and speak to no one. At least you would, hopefully, have had

World population = 5000 million
10% are queer = 500 million
Half are men = 250 million

Turned Down?

There are 249,999,999 others to choose from

Get Cruising!

Cruising Safely

Safer Sexy

some interesting conversations. Give yourself some brownie points for having had the guts to try.

When you get turned down, avoid taking it as a personal slight. There are many different reasons why a guy isn't interested. Often his reasons have nothing to do with you. He may have a boyfriend, he may have just broken up with his partner and not feel ready for sex with someone new. There's the possibility that he's insecure and feels you are too good for him. You might remind him of an ex-lover he wants to forget. He may have to get up early the next morning for an important business appointment. Perhaps he's tired or unwell, and has a lot of problems weighing on his mind. Most likely of all, you're simply not his type. He prefers a guy of a different age or physique. Maybe he only goes with skinny disco bunnies, hairy manual workers, middle-aged chubbies or black professionals.

Thankfully, sexual attraction is immensely varied and idiosyncratic. Whatever your appearance or personality, there are guys out there who'll fancy you. It's just a matter of finding them. That's why the best response to rejection is not to give up. Carry on cruising until you strike lucky. Sooner or later, you will.

Some guys set themselves up for rejection by having an off-putting cruising style. They come on too strong, or they have an unfriendly manner. Others persistently cruise men who are unlikely to be interested in them, perhaps because of a big difference in style, age or social background – and then wonder why they are so often turned down. If you find yourself locked into a cycle of rejection, it's important to stop and figure out what you're doing wrong. Change your cruising style. Try some new venues. Vary the type of guys you go for. See if you have more luck by sometimes waiting for men to approach you.

Rejection is never enjoyable, but it can be more bearable if it's done with tact and style. When a guy engages you in conversation or asks for a dance, even if you're not interested, accept his flattery and thank him. If you are happy to talk or dance for a few minutes, oblige him. Then excuse yourself. That way no one loses face.

Cruisewise safety

Cruising is usually very safe and trouble-free. But it can sometimes be risky. Wandering around secluded woodlands in the middle of the night, or going down dark alleys with a total stranger, does make us vulnerable to those who wish us harm. There are the dangers of getting beaten or raped by queer-bashers and attacked or robbed by a pick-up.

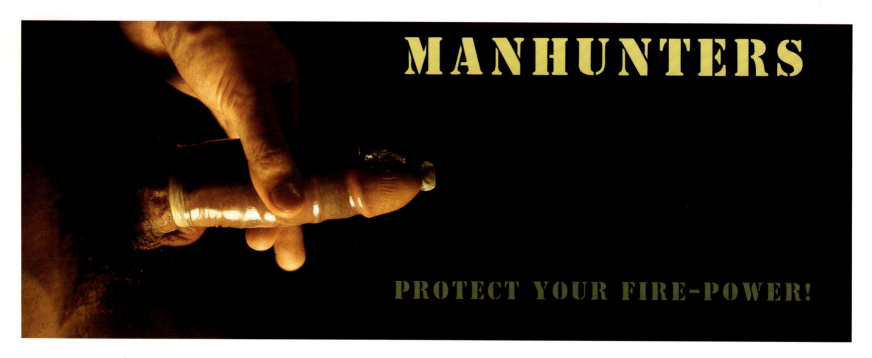

MANHUNTERS

PROTECT YOUR FIRE-POWER!

Although these things happen relatively rarely, they are ever-present possibilities. Fortunately, we can easily reduce the dangers by following the safe cruising code:

⚥ Carry a whistle with you at all times.

⚥ Don't go out with lots of cash or credit cards.

⚥ Stay alert and be aware of who is around you, especially behind you.

⚥ Steer clear of groups of loud and boisterous young straight men.

⚥ Walk with purpose and confidence, as if you know where you are going (even if you don't).

⚥ Wherever possible stick to busy, well-lit streets or parks or locations with other people nearby.

⚥ Whenever you feel threatened, walk where the light is brightest. Go to the curb so you can be seen better by passing motorists. Move to a place where there are other people, such as a store, bar or train station.

⚥ Avoid unfamiliar, isolated or dangerous areas, if you are drunk or stoned.

⚥ If you are followed and fear imminent attack, blow your whistle and scream for help.

⚥ In situations where you're assaulted, especially when you are outnumbered, try to run away as fast as you can, preferably to a crowded location where you can 'get lost' or summon assistance.

⚥ If you're cornered and can't escape, scream to scare off the bashers. If that doesn't work, act confident. Try talking while you walk away facing them. If the bashers attack you, act tough. Improvise a weapon. Clench your keys or a pen in your fist to make a short, blunt knife-like weapon. Aim for the

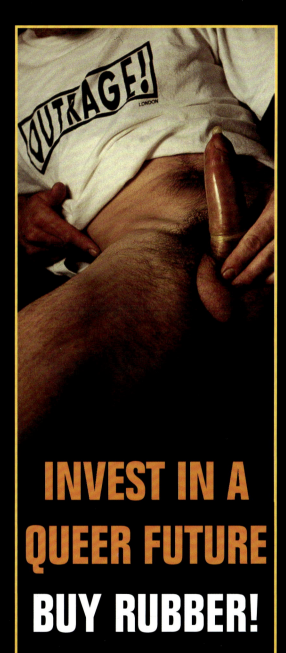

INVEST IN A QUEER FUTURE BUY RUBBER!

Cruising Safely
Safe pick-ups

most vulnerable point. Stab them in the eyes. If you cannot improvise a weapon, jab your fingers into their eye sockets. Run away as soon as you can.

⚥ If you see another guy being attacked, don't ignore him or run away. Go to his aid. If this is too dangerous, blow your whistle and scream to frighten off the attackers. Warn other people and ask for their help. If no one else is around, bang on nearby doors and windows to attract attention. Flag down passing cars and get the drivers to help. Telephone for the police and an ambulance. If the bashers flee in a car, note the car make, colour and registration number. As soon as feasible, write down a detailed description of the attackers. Give all this information to the police as soon as they arrive on the scene. If you do not feel able to trust the police, get your local lesbian and gay helpline to pass on this information on your behalf.

⚥ Gay bashers often target cruising grounds like parks and toilets. At the first sign of an anti-queer lynch mob, most guys scatter like chickens. This makes us vulnerable to being picked off one by one. Usually, there are several gay men and only two or three attackers. If all of us stayed together, and acted tough and confident, we would easily outnumber the queer-bashers and could probably scare them off. Better still we could bash back!

Next time you see a gang of bashers trying to lynch a queer, band together with all the other gay men and beat the shit out of the bastards. Then turn them over to the police. Make sure they're prosecuted, convicted and put behind bars.

Safe pick-ups

Compared to the drunken violence of many straight bars, gay venues are generally much safer and

Cruising Safely

friendlier. Gay men prefer to fuck guys, not fight them. We've got fewer sexual and emotional hang-ups compared with heteros. This makes it much easier for us to be open, intimate, giving and adventurous with strangers. While these are very positive attributes, they also put us at risk of attack from queer-bashers, and from psychos in our own community.

Not everything is rosy in the queer garden. Although we don't have the same level of pathological aggression as straight men, there are gay thieves, blackmailers, rapists, muggers and serial killers. However rare, they do exist.

It is unwise to allow the bulge in your jeans to override your commonsense. Protect yourself from danger when picking up new partners by taking precautions:

- Don't try to cruise or pick up guys if they have an unfriendly attitude, or if they are with other men who are not obviously gay.

- Keep your wallet in a pocket where it can't be lifted easily while you're cruising, picking up or having sex.

- When you decide to go home with a guy you've met for the first time, try to make sure that someone knows that you've gone with him. If you're in a bar, introduce him to a friend, bartender or doorman. If you have met the guy in the street or at a cruising ground, make sure another man notices him with you. Stop and ask a stranger for the time or a light. Make conversation with a fellow passenger or ticket collector on the train. Maybe you could call in briefly to see a friend or neighbour on the way home.

- It's safest to have first-time sex with a new partner in a house where other people are present. If you live alone, ask friends if you and your pick-up can stay the night at their home.

- When a guy invites you back to his house and you don't feel comfortable when you get there, trust your instincts. Make an excuse to go. Thank him for his time, and offer to meet him the next day. Then leave.

- Men who are into bondage scenes, where they get tied up, are very vulnerable. Never allow another man to tie you up unless you have previously introduced him to friends, and ideally not until you have seen him a few times and have satisfied yourself that he's safe.

- If you make contact with a guy via a telephone sex line, personal contact ad or dating service, do not agree to meet up with him without first getting his home phone number and discreetly ringing him back to confirm it is correct. Then, before you meet up with your new man, leave his number and the date, time and place of your planned meeting with a reliable friend. Avoid a rendezvous at his house or yours. Choose a neutral place, like a bar or cafe, where there are plenty of people around.

Avoiding arrest

Despite record levels of violent crime, some police officers prefer to spend their time harassing those of us who are engaged in harmless cruising and discreet sex. Heterosexuals fucking in lovers' lanes rarely get picked up by the police, but gay men caught having sex in obscure places nearly always get arrested. So we need to make sure we don't get caught:

- Don't have sex in any place where it might be visible to members of the public who may be offended and could call the police.

- Be on the lookout for police traps and surveillance operations; they often use unmarked cars and are not in uniform.

- Don't stand by and allow the police to pick off other gay men. Whenever you notice a police presence, carefully warn other cruisers – but do not make your actions too obvious, otherwise you might be arrested for obstructing the police. Later, inform your local lesbian and gay newspaper so it's readers can be warned.

- If you see a gay man being arrested for cruising, give him your telephone number and offer to testify on his behalf. Get contact numbers from other cruisers who are prepared to act as witnesses against the police.

- If you get arrested, never allow yourself to be represented by a local or police lawyer. Always get a lawyer who specialises in defending gay men, preferably a gay one.

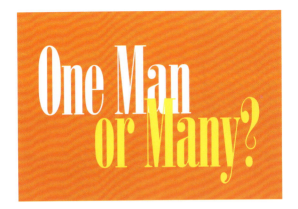

One Man or Many?

Needs and choices

Which is best? Falling in love and settling down with one special guy, or remaining single and enjoying the freedom to sleep with lots of different men? There isn't a right answer. It varies according to each individual's own needs and desires. Whatever your choice, there are pros and cons on both sides.

What validates sex is not eternal love, but mutual respect and erotic satisfaction. While sex with emotional commitment is a wonderful combination for some of us, sex can also be wonderful in its own right. Erotic enjoyment can be had with or without emotional involvement. It all depends on the preferences of the individual. What is right for one guy may not be right for another. Some prefer the security of sustained love and others prefer the novelty of new carnal conquests.

The only morality by which we ought to judge sexual relations is informed consent and mutual fulfilment. Whether these criteria are met in the context of an anonymous five-minute blow-job or a lifelong partnership is up to the guys concerned. If some of us choose to have lots of one-night stands, rather than a single permanent relationship, who has the right to say we are wrong? And if we get enjoyment from brief encounters, what right do others have to suggest they are unfulfilling?

Our personal sexual requirements vary enormously. There are guys whose sex drive craves release every day of the week, and those for whom once or twice a month is quite enough. At some point in our lives most of us want the sharing, commitment and support of a stable partnership. There can be other times when we long for the wild excitement of sexual abandon. Both are valid desires. We should all feel free to make whatever choices meet our needs and give us joy. Equally, everyone ought to feel able to change their choice when their needs change and when their happiness requires it.

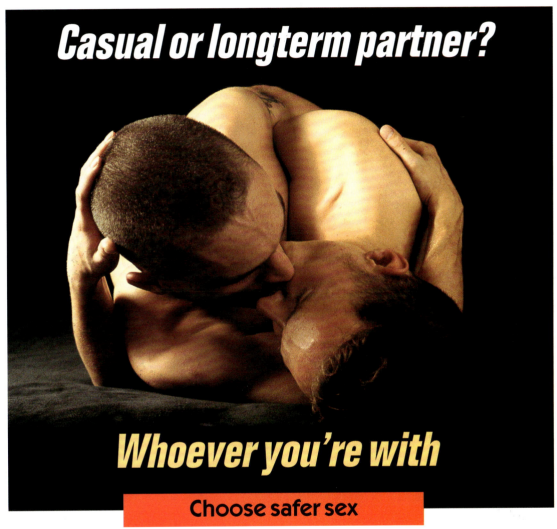

Casual or longterm partner?

Whoever you're with

Choose safer sex

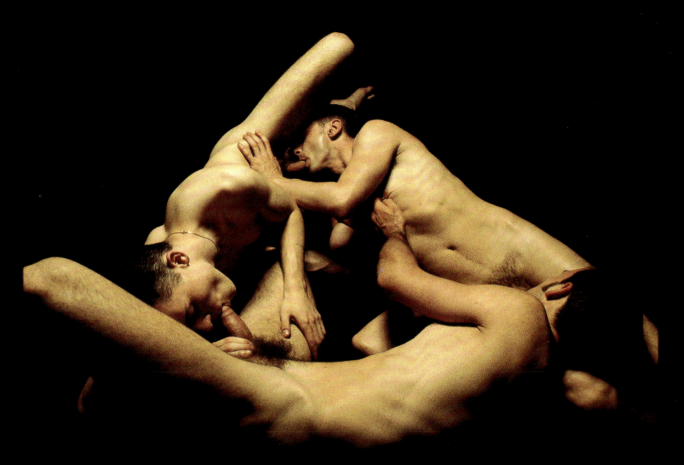

One Man or Many?
Playing the field

Settling down

It is true, of course, that for guys who are seeking the on-going commitment of a permanent relationship, endless affairs are sexually and emotionally unsatisfying. They can be very superficial, boring, and empty. One man can be looking for love while the other is interested only in lust and he can seem very selfish. A succession of one-night stands leaves many men feeling lonely and unvalued, and without emotional support. They may have no special, close friend to turn to and depend on in a time of personal crisis. Without a regular boyfriend, sex may be very intermittent. Sometimes you get it, sometimes you don't. As you get older, usually you don't. Occasionally, the urge to fuck gets out of control. Sexual conquest can then become an obsession and take over a guy's life, using up all his time and energy to the detriment of his work and friendships.

In contrast to short-lived liaisons, a committed relationship involves a deeper, more lasting intimacy. Guys get to know and understand each other to a degree that is impossible in a passing affair. A long-term partnership becomes a journey of mutual exploration and discovery out of which develop new levels of trust, sharing, empathy and support. This process of emotional bonding gives lovers a wonderful, reassuring feeling of deep personal strength and security which helps see them through the bad times as well as the good ones.

Needless to say, a stable relationship doesn't always indicate emotional health. For some, it might just be an expression of insecurity. For others, it may be little more than emotional dependency, or a convenient domestic arrangement. There isn't a necessary correlation between maturity and monogamy. There are relationships where partners have stayed together and remained faithful for years, but at the price of losing all sense of romance, passion, individuality and fulfilment.

Playing the field

Having multiple sexual partners is sometimes a second best substitute for a much desired, but unattained, longterm relationship. Alternatively, it may conceal a deeper emotional coldness and immaturity, including a fear of closeness, or anxiety about rejection. But not necessarily. Sleeping with lots of men may simply indicate a powerful and healthy libido, unhampered by guilt and hang-ups. It can sig-

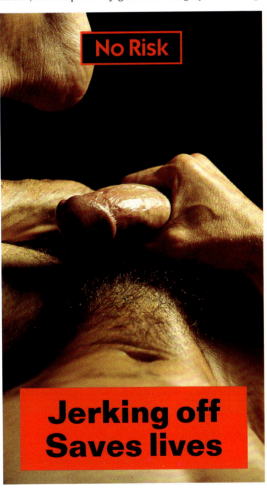

nify a strong sense of personal independence and self-reliance. Not everyone feels the emotional need for a relationship. Screwing with many men may signify a taste for sexual adventure. There are plenty of guys for whom the thrill of the chase, and the excitement of conquest or submission, is far more satisfying than the cosy comfort of a permanent commitment. Every new seduction is unique and this fact gives it an intense erotic charge that sex with a regular lover, no matter how enjoyable, can never replicate. The arousal produced by the anticipation of the unknown, and by the first touch of an unexplored body, is prodigious. It is precisely these feelings of newness, difference, uniqueness and adventure that make having sexual experiences with lots of men so exhilarating.

A wide range of erotic experience also has value in that it increases erotic skills; the result is that queers are good at sex. This has nothing to do with innate sexual prowess – it is a case of practice makes perfect. The larger number of sexual partners, compared to most straight guys, results in gay men having a generally higher level of erotic awareness and sophistication, and a greater degree of sexual confidence and satisfaction.

As in any activity, the more experience one has the more proficient one's technique becomes. Good sex, like good pair skating or tennis doubles, involves picking up tips from a process of accumulated experience with a range of different partners. Greater diversity in sexual encounters is bound to produce a more diverse range of sexual techniques.

You must make your own choice about whether you prefer one man or many. Whatever you decide, make sure it is a choice that fulfils your needs and happiness while also respecting the needs and happiness of others.

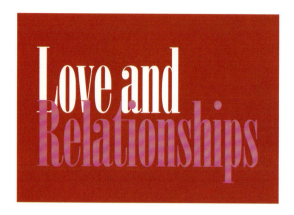

Love and Relationships

Sex is wonderful. Love is fabulous. Both together is out of this world. Being in love combines the physical joy of lust and sexual satisfaction with the enduring psychological and emotional pleasure of mutual support, intimacy, sharing, dependability, companionship and security.

There is no single, fixed model of relationship that suits everyone. It's up to you and your partner to explore and experiment to find the type of relationship that meets your needs best and gives you the most joy. Sometimes, this may involve going against social conventions. That's not such a bad thing. Why should we mimic the often flawed example of heterosexual marriage? All gay relationships break the rules of straight society. Men are not supposed to fall in love with each other. Having transgressed one rule, we should not be afraid, when necessary for our personal happiness, to transgress others.

Formulas for success

There is no way to guarantee a successful relationship, but you can increase the chances. The most enduring and satisfying love affairs tend to based on:

Compatibility

Being compatible is about more than great fucks. It also involves having personalities, lifestyles and non-sexual interests that click together. Although some common ground is necessary, compatibility doesn't mean partners must be identical. Differences are okay – providing they are complementary, and providing the partners are able to understand and accept each other's points of divergence. Indeed, very different guys can often hit it off as a couple if their differences complement each other or provide an interesting contrast. A guy who enjoys taking charge in a relationship, for example, usually gets on well with a guy who likes leaving the responsibilities to others. Likewise, if one partner is into mountaineering and the other is into architecture, each may find their partner's pursuit an interesting counter-balance to their own.

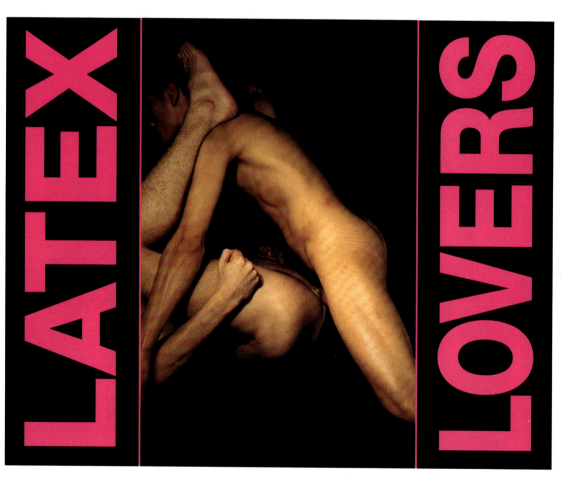

LATEX LOVERS

Love and Relationships
Formulas for success

Honesty

Telling the truth is always right. A lot of problems in relationships arise because partners are not open about their feelings. They fail to make clear their needs, desires, fears and hopes; this leads to unnecessary misunderstandings and conflicts. Bottling up feelings also often breeds frustration and resentment which later explode in sudden destructive rage. Being honest about the way you feel is sometimes painful, but it is essential if you want to face up to problems and resolve them. The discussion of difficulties can be made easier if you both take the trouble to create a supportive atmosphere where you know that telling the truth will be appreciated and not be regarded as a threat. With good communication, partners understand each other better. Tensions can be nipped in the bud. The bottom line is that there can be no genuine love without honesty. If lovers cannot trust each other, the basis of a meaningful committed relationship ceases to exist.

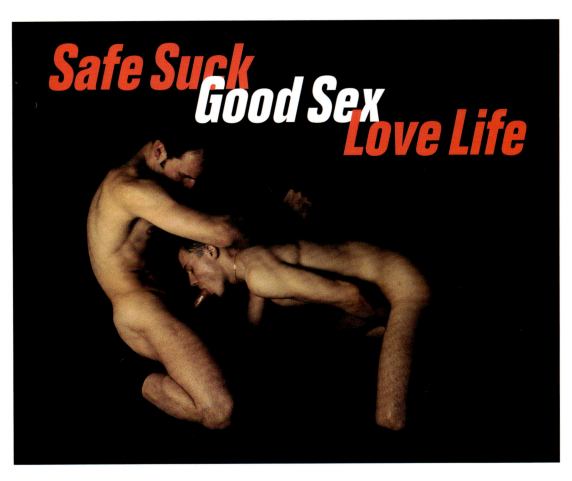

Mutual support

Sharing and mutual support are what makes an emotional commitment between two people worthwhile. Life's difficulties become easier to cope with when there is someone special who understands and cares. Supportiveness is, of course, about more than standing by one another through adversity, like a career setback or the death of a friend. It also involves sharing the joys, like a knitted sweater, a new home or receiving an award for community service. Without mutuality, relationships are doomed. One-sided, selfish affairs never work because they are draining and conflict builds up. A partner who makes all the effort while his mate contributes very little will feel used and dissatisfied.

The result: endless anger and arguments. In contrast, successful partnerships are based on a two-way exchange of support – each partner giving to the other, and having that giving reciprocated. This shared generosity becomes mutually reinforcing. It creates an upward expanding spiral of giving and receiving which emotionally enriches both partners and their relationship.

Flexibility

When we first fall in love, our happiness makes us want to preserve all those magic moments and feelings forever. We are reluctant to change. But nothing stays the same. Like everything else, relationships change over time. Partners develop and mature, sometimes unevenly. When a relationship grows, we need to be able to grow with it. That requires flexibility in our attitudes and behaviour. Instead of being stuck in our ways and refusing to budge, we need to adapt positively to changes. This means a bit of mutual give-and-take. An inability to adjust to a changing relationship is a recipe for conflict.

Safer Sexy
Love and Relationships

Autonomy

Sharing doesn't mean you have to surrender your individuality and do everything together. It's important that you both have your own private time and space. Avoid crowding and smothering your partner. It's often a sign of jealousy and insecurity, and it can leave him feeling overwhelmed and trapped. Being together all the time can result in couples getting on each other's nerves, which leads to irritability and arguments. Give yourselves an occasional break from each other. Maintain separate, as well as shared, friends and interests. Respecting your partner's autonomy helps sustain the diversity that keeps relationships strong and interesting. Don't try to deny or erase your differences or change his personality. You fell in love with him because of who he is. Don't try to change him into somebody else. To do so is insulting and can destroy the loveable idiosyncrasies which attracted you to him in the first place.

Creativity

After lovers have been together for a while, a relationship can easily become stale and predictable. Partners slip into a routine and take each other for granted. The result is boredom and discontent. To keep relationships feeling exciting and energizing needs a bit of creative thinking. It means maintaining a sense of spontaneity (going off together on a spur of the moment holiday), imagination (trying out new sexual experiences), surprise (giving him an unexpected party), variety (not having the same routine night after night), daring (sharing a passionate kiss on a crowded train), experimentation (taking him to a club you have never visited before), freshness (redecorating the house) and versatility (swopping sex roles).

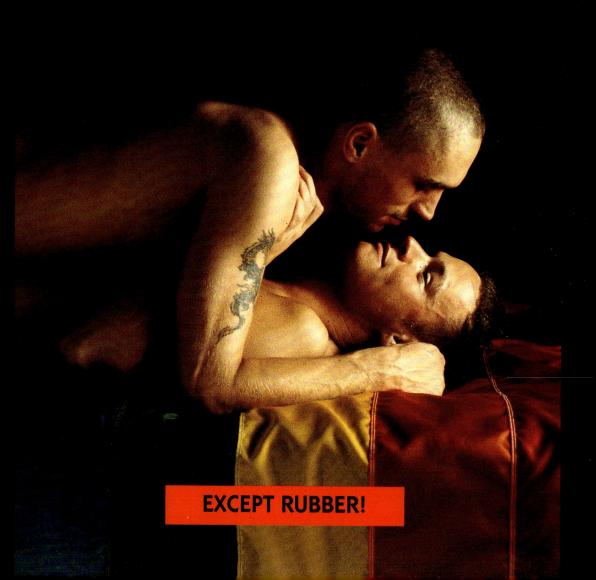

Don't let anything come between you and him...

EXCEPT RUBBER!

Open or closed relationships?

We aren't all the same. Our bodily and mental make-up is diverse. Consequently, different men have different sexual and emotional needs. The type of partnership that is appropriate for one guy is not necessarily appropriate for another. Some desire a longterm lover, plus the variety and adventure of additional periodic affairs. Others seek the familiarity and security of a single sexually exclusive relationship. These are all valid choices for those who make them, providing they are made with the free agreement of both partners. Having a secret affair behind a lover's back, without his agreement, is not right. It undermines trust. Without trust, no partnership can survive.

Sexual needs often change over time. What suits a man in his teens may not be right for him in middle-age. After years of sexual faithfulness, some guys in relationships need the release of an affair, even if only temporarily. They take a joint decision to have an open partnership where they can both have sex with other men. Conversely, those who have had a string of wild liaisons in their youth may yearn later for the stability of a closed partnership where they agree to only have sex with each other and with no one else.

Even among guys who want the sexual exclusivity of monogamy, not all of them can cope with, or live up to it. In the first couple of years of a relationship, when there is still lots of excitement and romance, sexual fidelity may be unproblematic. Later, however, as the thrill and freshness of a relationship wears off, routine and boredom can takeover. In these circumstances, monogamy is sometimes seen as a suffocating burden, and affairs are viewed as a source of zest and adventure.

Many gay men wisely make a clear distinction between sexual and emotional fidelity. If a guy has sex with a man other than his longterm partner, it need not necessarily devalue his commitment to the primary relationship. Sex is one thing and love is another. The two do not always go hand in hand.

Just as having an affair cannot automatically be equated with an absence of love for one's partner, sexual loyalty does not always coincide with the presence of love. Some couples stay faithful all their lives in boring, joyless partnerships. Others maintain satisfying asexual relationships. Many come to an arrangement to have minor affairs concurrently with their passionate lifelong relationship. They are able

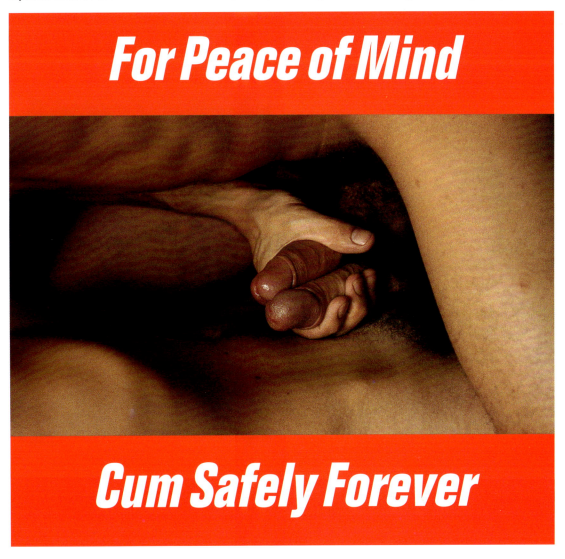

Safer Sexy
Love and Relationships

to cope with these affairs without any problem because their love is based on a lot more than sex. This means when they fuck other men it poses no threat to their mutual commitment.

It's up to you and your partner to decide jointly whether you want an open relationship or a closed one. Whatever you want, be honest. Make your needs and vulnerabilities known to your partner. Acknowledge his requirements and anxieties too. Remember that a partnership is a balance of rights and responsibilities. Come to an agreement which takes into account your feelings and his.

If you opt for an open relationship, involving the freedom to sleep with other men, it must be a negotiated decision based on mutual consent and with full awareness of the possible pitfalls.

For this type of relationship to work, both partners need to be able to overcome the possessive attitude that our lovers are our property. Loving someone is not the same as owning them. Good relationships are based on partners choosing to stay together because they respect and value each other, and not through the denial of freedom and trust.

Sexual jealousy is mostly an expression of low self-esteem and insecurity. A guy who does not regard himself very highly may fear he will be abandoned if his partner has sex with other men. Overwhelmed by the worry that his lover will meet someone better than him, he feels threatened and becomes very possessive. This reflects his sense of worthlessness and his anxiety about the loss of his partner to someone else. It also suggests that he sees sex as the main thing that holds a relationship together; that without an erotic hold over his partner there would be little to sustain their relationship.

An open relationship is disastrous when two guy's commitment to each other is ambiguous and superficial. It can work only if a partnership is strong and confident, and is held together by more than sex. Even then, partners who think they can cope with an

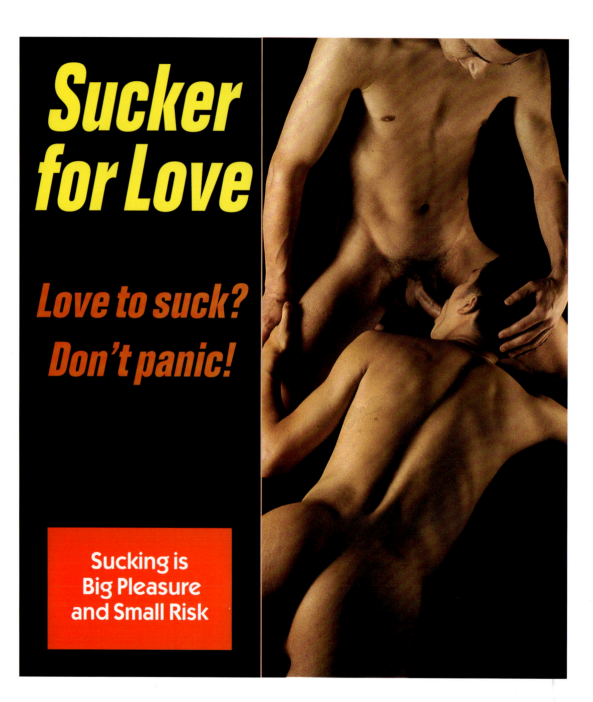

Sucker for Love

Love to suck? Don't panic!

Sucking is Big Pleasure and Small Risk

Love and Relationships
Breaking up

open relationship sometimes find it very threatening. If one partner has more sex, or gets to bed more glamorous men, the other partner may feel envious and resentful. And there's always bad timing – one partner may have a sexual fling when the other is expecting his attention.

It is important for couples in open relationships to agree rules which combine freedom with sensitivity. A man may be willing for his partner to have sex with other men, for example, but not feel comfortable about meeting the men he sleeps with. To diffuse the potentially threatening nature of open relationships, partners need to set parameters which respect their vulnerabilities and give them a sense of security. Possible rules include:

❦ Going out together must always end with returning home together.

❦ Sex with other men must be limited to (a) once-only encounters, (b) shared threesomes, or (c) periods when partners are separated due to work assignments, etc.

❦ Other sexual contacts must always be talked about openly (or never talked about).

❦ Partners having affairs must not stay out overnight.

❦ Another sexual partner must never be brought back to the house or introduced (or always brought back to the house and introduced).

❦ Liaisons with other men must be limited to certain nights of the week.

By devising ground rules like these, you can minimize friction and ensure that an open relationship operates in ways that you both agree, understand and feel comfortable with.

Dealing with difficulties

All relationships go through good and bad patches. It's unrealistic to expect perfect, trouble-free bliss forever. The most loving partners have disagreements occasionally. These can sometimes cause tension and conflict. Although often passing dramas, they may be symptomatic of deeper difficulties if they keep recurring on a regular basis.

The warning signs of a troubled relationship are:

❦ Frequent disagreements and rows.

❦ Increased irritability and bad moods.

❦ Repeated cancellation of planned dates.

❦ Ignoring a partner when out together with friends.

❦ Resistance to physical touch.

❦ Fewer pre-sex caresses and after-sex cuddles.

❦ Long bouts of silence and unresponsiveness to conversation.

❦ Less regular and more rushed sex.

❦ Excessive consumption of alcohol or drugs.

❦ Unexplained absences, or the non-return of phone calls.

Sometimes, these warning signs are staring us in the face, but we fail to recognize them. The feeling of being in love is wonderful and over-powering. It tends to make us very optimistic and forgiving. We always think the best of our partner and are reluctant to admit his shortcomings. The fear of loss and loneliness makes us want to believe he still loves us. As a result, we fail to see the relationship as it really is. Evidence of problems are blocked out of our mind and erased from our memory. Bad behaviour is rationalized as unintentional or inconsequential.

When the warning signs appear, the priority is to recognize and tackle the underlying problems in the relationship. Common problems range from the petty to the serious: selfishness (he eats your share of the chocolate fudge), laziness (failure to do household chores), lifestyle differences (he wants to party, you prefer to stay at home), workaholism (concentrating on career to the neglect of a relationship), domination (lack of respect for your privacy and autonomy), sexual incompatibility (he wants sex in ways you don't enjoy), chemical dependence (drug or alcohol abuse sparking unpredictable mood swings), illicit affairs (breaking the agreement to be monogamous).

It's so important to confront a difficulty the moment it arises, not leave it to fester and grow. Be ready to talk with your partner, choose a place with privacy, a time when you both have no pressing engagements. Remind him of your love for him. Let him know you feel there is a relationship problem. Spell out your reasons. Express your discontent and unhappiness. Be straightforward and firm, but tactful. Give him time for his response. Avoid aggression, threats, guilt-tripping and humiliation. Stay calm and reasoned. Make it clear you want to save the relationship, not end it. Offer him options, not ultimatums. Listen to his feelings. Make a shared agreement to deal with the problem.

Breaking up

Relationships are a risky business. They don't always work out. But without a willingness to take the risk of failure, no love affair can ever succeed.

All relationships have a start and a finish. Most gay men tend to have several significant relationships over the course of their lifetime. What is important is the quality of a relationship, not the length of its duration. Many gay lovers pack more thrills and

Safer Sexy
Love and Relationships

affection into a twelve month partnership than some husbands and wives muster in years of marriage. A short fulfilling relationship is surely better than a long dull one. No one should be afraid of splitting up when a relationship ceases to bring them satisfaction. Instead, it should be seen as a positive opportunity to remove a cause of pain and to give oneself the freedom to develop in new and happier directions.

It's a fact of life that people change over time. Lovers sometimes diverge. They develop different interests, attitudes, lifestyles and sexual tastes. Often these changes are manageable, but sometimes they are impossible to cope with. When a damaged relationship does not respond to attempts to put it right, the mature reaction is not to grin and bear it, but to make a clean break and move on to something better that will bring you happiness – and allow him freedom to find new happiness also.

Of course, no previously valued relationship should ever be ended without an attempt to save it. If you are feeling grief and misery, it is important to identify the causes and discuss them frankly with your partner. Try to agree a plan of action to solve the problem. A solution may take time. Give it a chance. If there is no significant improvement after a reasonable length of time, let him know your patience is running out. Set a timetable for some positive changes.

When all efforts to solve relationship difficulties come to nothing, it's time to think long and hard about your future together. Write a list of pros and cons. Ask yourself: Am I prepared to put up with this situation? Is our relationship worth the difficulties? Do the advantages outweigh the disadvantages? Would I feel happier with him or without him?

If you decide to split, think it over carefully for a few days to make sure you have made the right decision. Then tell your partner to his face. Explain your feelings and reasons truthfully, but with sensitivity. Avoid being unnecessarily hurtful. Whatever has happened in the past, try to reach an amicable agreement to go your own separate ways. A bitter ending is emotionally corrosive and takes much longer to heal. If you want to remain friends, tell him so. If you would prefer no further contact, make that clear also.

To help yourself get over a traumatic bust up:

⚤ Recognise that although you miss him, you can get by without him.

⚤ Avoid thinking you could have saved the relationship 'if only' you had acted differently. What's done is done. You can't change the past. Focus on future happiness.

⚤ Remember, if the relationship really had been wonderful, it would have survived. If you had been right for each other, you would still be together.

⚤ Splitting up is not the end of your love life. There are plenty of wonderful men out there. Some are much better than he could ever be. Look on finishing an old relationship as an opportunity to start a new and more rewarding one.

⚤ If you feel morbid and depressed, don't spend long periods at home alone. Get out and get active. Keep your mind occupied to prevent gloomy thoughts. You may not yet feel ready for cruising and clubbing, but you can visit friends and have them round for dinner.

⚤ Think of all the things you wanted to do but never did because he was around. Go out and do them. Have that holiday he always vetoed. Try sex acts that he would never do.

⚤ Work-out at the gym or take up a sport to burn up your anger and resentment. Hard physical activities also produce lots of 'happy hormones' which can help restore your sense of mental and emotional well-being.

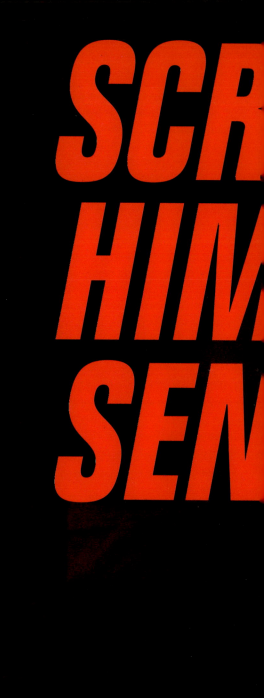

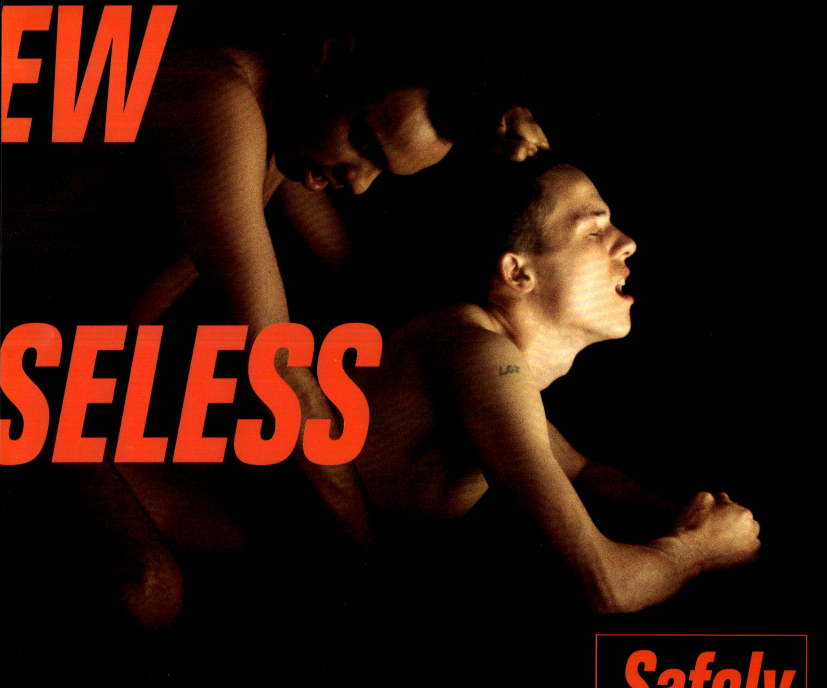

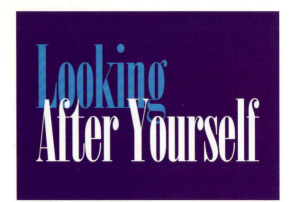

Looking After Yourself

Safety first

If you tend to worry over every minute or theoretical risk of giving or getting HIV, don't! It's not necessary. Sensible precautions are justifiable; paranoia is not. Finger cuts, mouth ulcers, razor nicks, and bleeding gums are extremely unlikely ways of passing on the virus. They pale into insignificance compared to the dangers of unprotected fucking.

However, if you still feel anxious, and really want absolutely to minimize your risk while maximizing your body care and freshness, then there are several practical safety hints you can follow:

Cover sores, cuts and rashes

If you have any open sores, cuts or abrasions on your body, do not get another man's cum, blood, serum, piss or shit on them – and don't let your blood get into another man's body. To be safe, cover any wounds with a waterproof band-aid before having sex. Guys with skin complaints like eczema or psoriasis should keep the affected area under wraps and well away from their partner's body fluids, especially if the skin is raw, cracked or weeping.

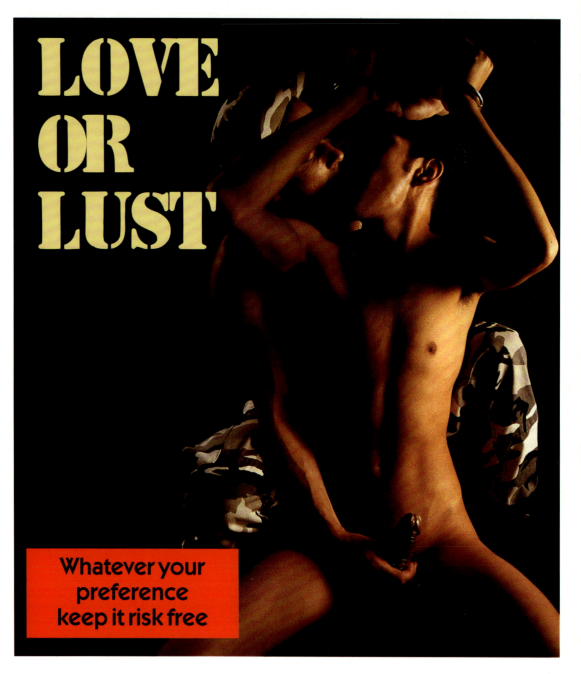

LOVE OR LUST

Whatever your preference keep it risk free

Looking After Yourself
Safety first

Check your mouth

From time to time, some of us get mouth ulcers and bleeding gums or sometimes bite our tongue or cut our gums on sharp bits of food. Any open wound inside the mouth may increase the risk of HIV infection if another guy's body fluids get into your mouth, although this risk is a very small one. However, if you feel the need to be extra safe, whenever you notice sores or wounds in your mouth, especially with visible blood, it's best to avoid wet kissing, cock sucking and licking arse until they have healed. That will protect both you and your partner if either of you have HIV.

Douche and enema care

Too much use of a douche, or enema, to wash out your arse before being fucked, licked or fisted is not a good idea. Although it may make you feel clean, it doesn't remove all the germs and can spread them to the outside of your arse. This might make your partner more likely to pick up an infection, such as hepatitis or ameobiasis, if he fingers or licks you around the butt. Besides, using a douche or enema can wash away good bacteria which are necessary for a healthy arse. It also destroys the natural moist lining inside your butt. This might make you slightly more prone to friction damage during fingering or fucking.

Occasional use of a douche or enema with a rounded, smooth nozzle is okay. Apply some lubrication to ease it inside you. Only use plain water. Disinfectants and antiseptics can harm the lining of the arse. Always shower thoroughly after an enema or douche to clean away germs from the outside of your butt.

Avoid douches and enemas with sharp or rough nozzles. These can cause tears and abrasions to the delicate tissues inside the arse-hole, which may increase the danger of HIV. Never share douches or enemas with a partner, as this could transfer infection. Trying to wash cum out of your arse after fucking without a condom is useless. It offers no protection against HIV and it may raise your risk of infection if the lining of your butt is damaged.

Shave with care

Some guys swoon over a smooth, just-shaved face. But take care.

∂∂ Wet shaving, with foam and a hand razor, can result in tiny cuts. If you nick your skin while shaving, don't fret. Just avoid getting another guy's body fluids on the wound.

∂∂ Cuts during wet shaving can

SEX WITH SAFETY = SEX WITHOUT FEAR

Safer Sexy
Looking After Yourself

leave blood on the blade. This makes it risky to share razors with your partner; you could transfer blood from one guy to another. So, make sure you both have your own razors and avoid sharing them.

🔹 Men who are prone to shaving nicks, or who get a bad skin reaction from wet razors, could try using an electric shaver or a beard removing gel.

Brush teeth gently

Be gentle when cleaning your teeth, especially if you plan to go out cruising or on a date. Hard brushing or flossing can occasionally cause gum abrasion and bleeding. The danger is *very* small, but this may make you slightly vulnerable to giving or getting HIV if you suck off a guy, or deep kiss a man who also has cuts and blood in his mouth.

🔹 If you suffer from bleeding gums, have them checked out and treated by your dentist.

🔹 Sharing a toothbrush is not safe. Get your own and keep it to yourself.

🔹 Use a soft toothbrush.

🔹 Avoid brushing your teeth immediately before or after sex. If you really need to clean your teeth before jumping into bed, try rubbing them with toothpaste on your finger or vigorously swilling some mouthwash.

🔹 Restrict flossing your teeth to times of the day when you are least likely to have a sexual rendezvous.

Clip and file fingernails

Sharp and broken fingernails are neither stylish nor safe. They look tacky and can tear condoms. They can also cause scratches and cuts when jerking off or when fingering or fisting a guy's arse.

To prevent damage, clip your nails short and file them smooth. Gently sand down any rough skin. It will leave your fingers feeling soft and sensual, and allow them to get on with lots of hard-core action without risk.

Remove jewellery

Watches, rings and bracelets sometimes have sharp edges which can rip condoms and graze skin while jerking off, putting on rubbers or finger and fist-fucking. To be safe, take them off before getting down to passion.

Swapping and sharing earrings or other body piercing jewellery may be risky when the piercings are new or when the skin around them is cracked – this could transfer blood. If you want to swop, sterilize the piercing jewellery by boiling it vigorously or by soaking it in strong disinfectant.

Getting fresh

The feel and smell of a freshly showered or bath-soaked body is a great turn-on for many of us, although some guys prefer natural body aromas. It is also good hygiene. Although it is not an essential part of safer sex, taking a shower before jumping into bed is a smart idea if you plan to run your lips and fingers around each other's dicks and arses. You don't necessarily know where your partner has been or what he has been up to just before he met you. Showering or bathing together, can make a very erotic prelude to sex. Being rubbed down and lathered up under a jet of tingling water gets many guys hot and horny, *fast!*.

Showering is also a good way to finish sex – washing off potentially infectious body fluids. Sex is

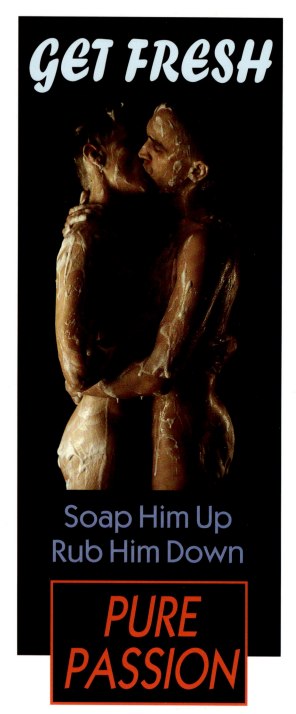

GET FRESH

Soap Him Up
Rub Him Down

PURE PASSION

Looking After Yourself
Turn-offs and remedies

messy. It can leave minute traces of cum and shit on your body which can easily be accidentally picked up with your fingers or lips. So, if you want to be extra safe and feel refreshed, shower before and after sex.

Turn-offs and remedies

There are lots of sexy things that turn us on. There are also some very unsexy things that turn us off. Many of these relate to personal hygiene. Even really handsome men can ruin their looks, and put off other guys if they are dirty and unkempt. It can signal that they don't care and can't be bothered. That's not very alluring. For most of us, fresh-scrubbed looks and smells are highly erotic stimuli. They enhance sex appeal, giving even ordinary-looking guys an added glow and zest. Looking and smelling clean gives your partner the confidence to tongue and kiss all over your body, including those hygiene-sensitive areas, such as your arse, dick, feet and arm-pits. He might be reluctant to do that if he thinks you're not clean – and you'll miss out on some exquisite erotic delights such as a sexy arse-licking or toe-sucking.

Making sure you are clean and fresh is about looking after yourself and looking your best. To take good care of your appearance is a sign of self-esteem and self-confidence. These can be very attractive attributes. However, while it is good to be clean, it is not good to be obsessive about it. A hint of fresh, natural body smells can be quite arousing; sometimes more so than a body drowned in aftershave and deodorants. Some guys are into really dirty, sleazy sex. They get turned on by filth and foul smells. That's fine if it is a shared desire. However, most of us find cleanliness sexier.

The most commonly cited turn-offs are: bad breath, greasy hair, smelly feet, nose bogeys, ear wax, dirty teeth, stale sweat, dandruff, furry tongue,

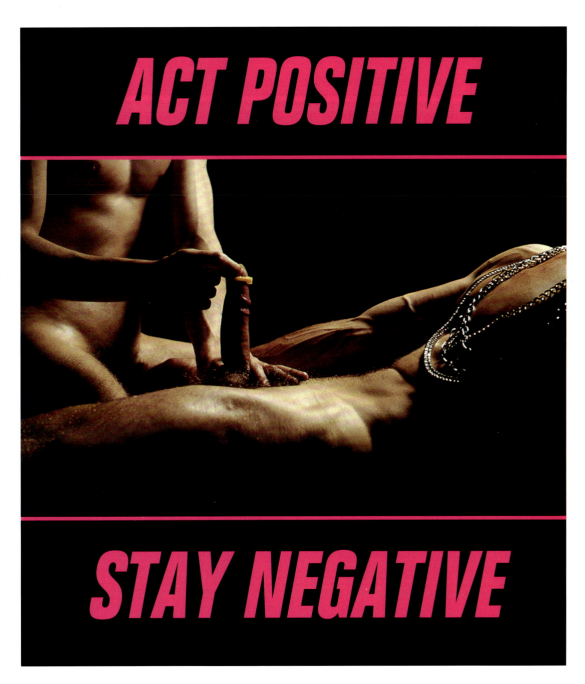

Safer Sexy
Looking After Yourself

oily skin, cheesy dick, grubby finger-nails, pimples, ear and nose hairs, and shit or toilet paper around the arse.

We can eliminate nearly all of these turn-offs. Some, such as particular skin problems, may be beyond our immediate control, but most can be quickly and easily remedied. Before you go out bar-hopping or to a boyfriend's house for dinner, check yourself over.

The three big turn-offs that most guys find most off-putting are:

Bad breath

The causes of bad breath are dirty teeth, gum disease, tooth decay, smoking, excessive alcohol, over-eating, stale garlic and strong spices and, in particular, stomach and intestinal disorders. These gut disorders are the main cause of really foul smelling breath and are usually related to prolonged stress, infection, food allergies or to the digestive system not working properly.

To prevent bad breath:

- Brush your teeth morning and night. Try rinsing out your mouth with a disinfectant mouthwash before sex.
- Give up smoking.
- Moderate your intake of alcohol and food.
- Avoid garlic and spicy dishes if you plan to go out cruising or out on a date.
- Reduce your stress. Find ways to relax during the week – gentle music, regular exercise, meditation.
- Avoid foods that can cause an allergic reaction.
- Get medical treatment for dental and digestive problems.
- Drink lots of water. Chew gum.

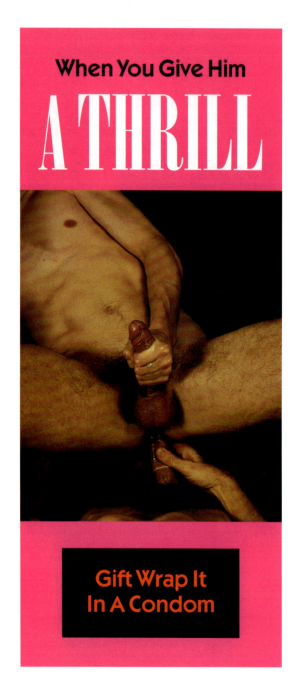

When You Give Him A THRILL

Gift Wrap It In A Condom

Stale sweat

Fresh sweat can be very sexy. Stale sweat isn't (unless you are into dirty sex). Shower every day and, if you love the smell and feel of a fresh body, shower before you have sex. Avoid strong under arm deodorants and anti-perspirants. They are bad for the skin and often have a bitter, metallic taste. This can ruin the passionate frenzy of a guy licking out your arm-pits. Choose a natural deodorant or a scented talc. It is kinder on your skin and his tongue.

Cock-cheese

Guys who are uncut (uncircumsized) experience the build up of a whitish, cheesy-smelling substance called 'smegma'. While a light whiff can be quite a turn-on, strong or stale cock-cheese is definitely a no-no for most guys. If you have a foreskin, be sure to pull it back and clean under it every day.

Healthy queer

Being gay is fabulous. Wild clubbing and cruising. New friends and lovers. Plenty of guys and sex.

The joy of accepting our sexuality and sharing it with others is a great liberation. However, being gay can sometimes involve a fast-track lifestyle that is very demanding: partying all weekend, late-night cruising, and pillow-talk into the small hours. Then there are the ups and downs of relationships, including the traumas of a broken heart.

All these pressures can take their toll. That's why it is vital to look after ourselves. Taking care helps make us feel and look healthier. With a healthy glow, we feel better about ourselves, and other guys find us more attractive.

Make the right choice. Live a healthy queer lifestyle.

Looking After Yourself
Healthy queer

Food for life

Food is the fuel of life. Eating badly deprives our bodies of essential nutrients. This makes us more vulnerable to sickness, and it does ghastly things like ruining our complexion.

A nutritious diet, on the other hand, maximizes our chances of staying healthy and looking good. It gives us the energy we need for rooting and rogering. The healthy eating code is:

- Drink less alcohol.
- Have regular well-balanced meals.
- Eat more fresh fruit, vegetables and wholegrains.
- Eat less meat, sugar, fat, processed food.
- Take a multivitamin supplement every day.

Sweet dreams

Relaxed and regular sleep is necessary to refresh and recharge our minds and bodies. Without it, we end up feeling tired, confused, run-down, and prone to infections like flu, spots and cold sores. And, we get that awful drawn, puffy-eyed look.

So listen, faggot! Get enough sleep to ensure that you wake up looking fresh, and feeling relaxed and energized. Don't party night after night without a break. If you miss one night's sleep, make it up the next night (or take an afternoon nap). That way, you'll look your best and be on top form if the man of your dreams suddenly walks into your life.

Work it, boy!

Suppleness, stamina, strength and sexiness; a fit body looks good to the eye and feels good to the touch. In bed, it can manoeuvre into all kinds of exotic sex positions, and sustain hard-core action

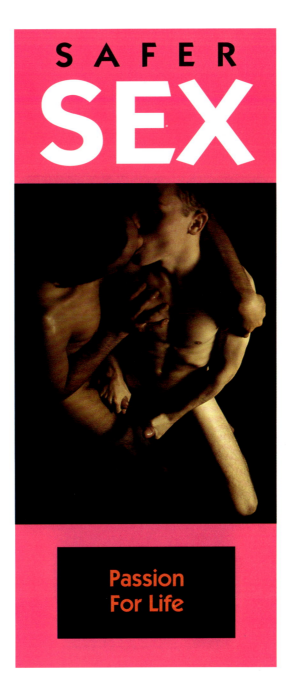

longer and stronger. A healthy physique is also better able to resist infection than a weak, run-down one. Regular exercise helps protect against illness by releasing lots of disease-fighting white cells into the bloodstream. It can help relieve stress and depression by flooding the brain with 'happy hormones', which give some guys a natural high.

To get your body hard and healthy, and your mind happy and horny, try a workout a couple of times a week at the gym. Or try a 20 minute early-morning workout at home using simple, weight-free exercises like push-ups, squats, back arches, knee lifts and stomach crunches. Alternatively, swim, jog or bike ride vigorously twice a week for an hour. You'll feel better, and look good too!

Cool out

When we're relaxed and at ease, it shows. We look radiant, feel good, and have an easygoing manner. Stress and anxiety have the opposite effect. Our body produces immune-suppressing hormones which increase our likelihood of sickness. We may also look terrible, be difficult to get on with, and could even lose our interest in sex. That plays havoc with relationships. Don't put up with stress:

- Avoid anxiety-provoking situations.
- Pace yourself and do not take on too many responsibilities.
- Communicate your feelings and express your emotions; don't bottle them up inside.

If you are stressed out, take time to unwind and relax. Do some deep breathing exercises, yoga or meditation. Try listening to serene, calming music. Have a massage, workout or sauna. Watch something funny on TV or get a slapstick classic out on video to get yourself laughing and happy.

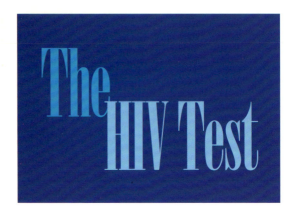

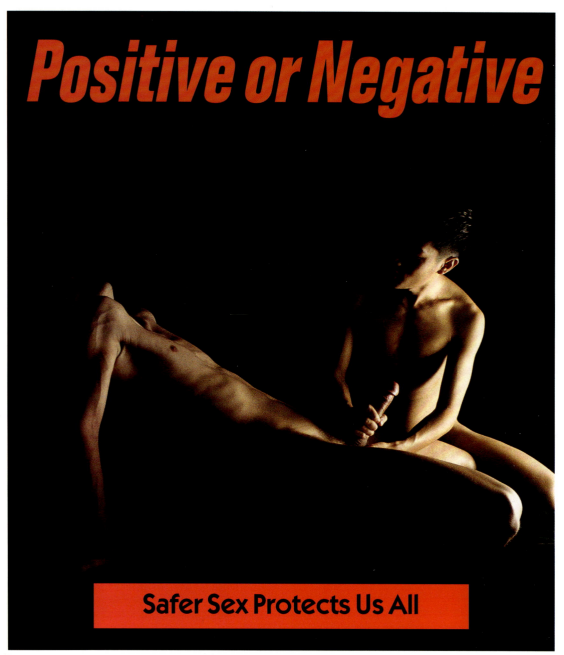

Safer Sex Protects Us All

The HIV Test

Getting tested for HIV is an option that some of us choose and some of us reject. It all depends on our own particular needs and circumstances. Whatever your decision, it's important to understand fully the implications of taking the test.

The 'HIV test' is a test for antibodies. When a guy is infected with HIV, his immune system produces specific antibodies to attack it. These antibodies stay in the blood indefinitely and can be identified in the test.

The HIV test shows whether or not any antibodies to HIV are present. If they are – a positive result – it is evidence that the person has been infected with HIV and is almost certainly still infectious. Such people are said to be 'HIV positive'. If no antibodies are detected – a negative result – this usually means the person has not been infected. These people are referred to as being 'HIV negative'.

However, it takes the body several weeks from the date of infection to develop detectable levels of HIV antibodies. This is sometimes called the 'window of infection' period and normally ranges from one to three months, although it can occasionally be as long as six months. During this period, a person could be infected with the virus and be infectious, but show no evidence of antibodies and register a

The HIV Test
To test or not?

negative result. Because of the delay in the appearance of antibodies, if you decide to take the HIV test, it's a good idea to wait until at least three months after the date you think you may have been at risk of infection. Even then, if you get a negative result it may be advisable to have a second test six months after the possible date of infection, just in case you are one of the small number of people who take longer than three months to produce noticeable amounts of antibodies.

The HIV test is almost 100% accurate but not foolproof. There are a number of safeguards to protect against errors. A 'false positive', which wrongly indicates the presence of antibodies, is usually uncovered and corrected by the practice of double-checking all positive results and repeating the test using a different method. A 'false negative', which mistakenly records the absence of antibodies, is normally rechecked if a person has a history of unsafe sex with HIV-positive partners or if they have symptoms associated with AIDS illnesses. This rechecking may involve a repeat antibody test or a special HIV antigen test which looks directly for the virus.

If you decide to get tested, it is recommended to go to a sexually-transmitted diseases (STD) clinic (also called a Genito-Urinary Medicine (GUM) clinic) rather than your local doctor. Clinic staff have specialist training and up-to-date knowledge about HIV. Their counsellors can give you expert advice and support in the event that your test is positive.

Compared to local doctors, clinics have stricter rules about confidentiality and non-disclosure of patient's records. This could be important if your ever apply for a mortgage, or medical insurance (companies may write to your local physician to ask whether you have had a HIV test and, if so, what the result was). They will often discriminate against applicants who've taken a test, even if the result was negative.

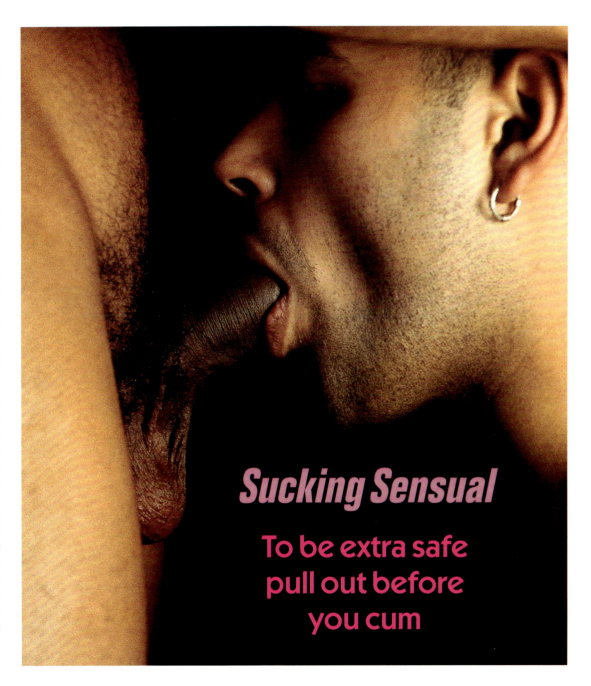

Sucking Sensual
To be extra safe pull out before you cum

The HIV Test — **Safer Sexy**

To test or not?

The drawbacks

If you are considering taking the HIV test, think seriously about its limitations:

🍆 A positive result does not show when, or if, you will later go on to become sick with AIDS.

🍆 Testing negative is not a guarantee that you aren't infected. If you have only recently contracted the virus, the antibodies may not show up in the test and you may register as a false negative.

🍆 Given that HIV is still incurable, getting tested is of little value as there is no truly effective and lasting treatment for those who test positive.

🍆 Most guys react to a positive result by feeling much more devastated than they expected. It usually provokes extreme anxiety and depression. This can further strain the immune system. You therefore need to ask yourself the following questions: Could I cope with the trauma of a positive result? How would it affect my partner and our relationship? Do I have enough close friends to give me the support I may need?

🍆 The mere fact of taking an HIV test, irrespective of the result, can lead to insurance and mortgage companies refusing cover or charging much higher premiums. If you test positive, you could be refused employment or housing, and you will be denied entry to some countries to holiday, study or work.

🍆 If you test HIV positive and people find out, you could face prejudice and abuse from your family, neighbours or work colleagues. This is likely to put you under additional stress, which may trigger serious sickness.

The advantages

Despite these drawbacks, there are several reasons why it may be beneficial to take the HIV test:

🍆 If you are very worried about being HIV positive, and worrying is making you ill, you could benefit from taking the test and clarifying your HIV status. Knowing the truth may be preferable to the anxiety and ill-health caused by the uncertainty. But think about it carefully. Are you absolutely sure that discovering you are HIV positive would cause you less worry than not knowing?

🍆 If you have HIV and get sick, being aware that you are HIV positive might assist the early diagnosis of your illness as being HIV-related. That could mean that doctors are able to begin treatment more quickly. In contrast, if no one knows that you have HIV, it might take doctors longer to realize that your symptoms are due to HIV infection.

🍆 It may be safer for your health to know if you are HIV positive. Then you can make sure you avoid exposure to potentially risky things like sun-beds, live vaccines, undercooked meats and disease-bearing animals.

🍆 Having an HIV test can help 'concentrate the mind'. It provides an opportunity for many of us to take on HIV as a personal issue for the first time. A test can also act as a catalyst for the adoption of less risky sexual practices: those of us who test positive often choose safer sex out of a desire not to pass the virus on to others, those of us who test negative often choose safer sex out of a desire to stay that way.

🍆 Guys who know they have the virus can benefit from regular medical monitoring. While HIV can't be cured yet, it can increasingly be managed and controlled, at least for a while. A growing number of medical treatments are able to delay the

---

HIV is no barrier to falling in love

Ignorance is!

Fight the fear with the facts

LOVE MEN WITH HIV

The HIV Test
To test or not?

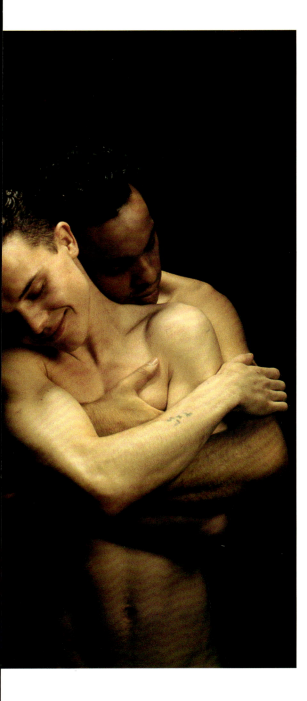

development of AIDS illnesses and reduce the frequency and severity of their occurrence. Crucial to the effectiveness of these 'early intervention' treatments is knowledge of a person's HIV status and the on-going monitoring of their immune system. This is a strong argument in favour of taking the test. It's an argument that will grow even stronger as more effective treatments come on stream and offer the prospect of improving the quality of life, and the survival time, of people with HIV.

※ For some of us, knowing our HIV status is a question of self-empowerment. Knowledge is power. If we test positive, we can make more informed decisions about options and priorities for the years ahead. It means we can actively plan for our future, rather than simply waiting for HIV to suddenly, without warning, strike us ill. This prior knowledge gives some of us much greater confidence. We feel in control of HIV, rather than it being in control of us.

※ If you take the test and the result is positive, there are constructive self-help things you can do to delay and reduce your chances of getting seriously sick. By taking good care of yourself and living a healthier lifestyle it's possible to strengthen your immune system and its ability to resist HIV. Useful do-it-yourself initiatives to build up your physical and psychological strength include meditation, mental imagery, nutritional supplements, regular sleep and exercise, stress limitation, and reduced consumption of cigarettes, alcohol and other recreational drugs.

Of course, everyone ought to be health-conscious. However, it's often the experience of taking the test that jolts many of us into looking after ourselves better. Some of us only make health-enhancing changes to our lives once we know we have HIV. Testing HIV positive and realizing we are vulnerable to life-threatening illnesses can be the catalyst for a switch to a healthier lifestyle; this switch may, indeed, significantly improve our survival prospects.

※ If you are in a longterm, committed relationship, you may look on testing as a safer sex strategy. You could choose to get tested with your partner. If you both have negative results, you might decide to cease practising safer sex with each other. Depending on whether you have an open or closed relationship, you may agree either to not have sex with any other man, or to have only safer sex with guys other than your lover. This decision – to give up safer sex if both of you test negative – is understandable, but risky. It assumes that the test result was accurate, and that neither of you was recently infected. It also depends on both of you sticking to your commitment to never have unsafe sex with other people. That's possible for some, but not for all. It's taking a lot on trust. About half the gay men who have contracted HIV got it unwittingly from a regular partner. Some guys in committed relationships have occasional flings and some get infected through unsafe sex during those brief affairs. They then inadvertently pass the virus to their lover. If you and your partner take the HIV test, get negative results, and want to abandon safer sex with each other, you need first to ask these questions: What happens if you or your partner has an affair and gets screwed without a condom? Or the condom breaks? Would he tell you? Would you tell him? How would that disclosure affect your relationship?

These are just some of the issues to consider before taking an HIV test. Whatever you decide, and whatever the result if you do take the test, choose safer sex to protect yourself and the men you love. HIV is stoppable, and you can be one of the people who helps stop it.

Preventable Diseases and Conditions

To have a long and enjoyable sex life, we need to look after our sexual health. This means adopting safer sex to prevent not only HIV, but other sex-related diseases as well. It also means identifying and getting treatment for illnesses such as testicular cancer which, although they are not transmitted sexually, can adversely affect our ability to have sex and may even jeopardize our lives. Some guys can have a sexually-transmitted disease without being aware of it. Either they show no obvious symptoms, or they fail to recognize the signs. Nevertheless, they can pass on the infection to others, including you. Checking your body for signs of infection once a week makes good sense. When you have a new sexual partner, it is advisable to check more regularly. Being on the lookout for infection ensures prompt recognition and treatment. This can save you a lot of discomfort, and the embarrassment of passing on an infection to someone else. It lessens the likelihood of permanent harm and minimizes the disruption to your sex life.

Because it's possible to have an infection without any noticeable symptoms, it's a sensible precaution to have a regular six monthly check-up at a sexually-transmitted diseases (STD) clinic, particularly if you've had unsafe sex, or sex with several different partners. If you are diagnosed with a sexually-related disease, always make sure you and your partner are treated at the same time to prevent reinfection. Sex-acquired diseases are not inevitable. They are not the 'necessary price' of a gay lifestyle. All the serious infections are preventable. Some of the less dangerous ones, such as glandular fever, are difficult to prevent. However, they are not very common and they clear up with treatment or of their own accord; they cause no longterm danger to health.

Fucking without a rubber is how the vast majority of sexually-transmitted diseases are spread. It's much more risky than any other sexual activity. Although arse-fingering, prick-sucking and butt-kissing can pass on diseases, they're much less risky than unprotected screwing. Using a condom every time you fuck massively decreases your chances of getting or giving HIV, or any other sex-related diseases.

HIV is by far the most dangerous disease that is transmitted through sex. It's mainly contracted by fucking without a condom. There is no cure for HIV. It can lead to AIDS and is often fatal. HIV is, however, totally avoidable. It is avoided through practising safer sex.

Apart from HIV, all other sexually-transmitted diseases are either non-fatal or curable except hepatitis B which can sometimes cause death due to liver failure or liver cancer. Hepatitis B is, however, preventable by means of a very effective vaccine.

Syphilis and gonorrhoea are two other very serious infections, but providing they are treated swiftly they do not cause lasting harm. If left untreated for many years, however, they can result in grave ill-health and sometimes death.

Other sexually-transmitted diseases may variously cause pain, itching or fatigue, but they are not life-threatening. Nevertheless they are best avoided as they can be damaging and may put the immune system under stress which is very dangerous if you already have HIV. Infections that are normally fairly harmless may further undermine your immune defenses by activating the more rapid replication of the virus.

It is of course important to keep the risk of HIV and other sexually-transmitted diseases in perspective. Everything we do in life has risks. Crossing the road, going swimming and using electrical gadgets can all be dangerous. However, we don't stop these activities because of the theoretical risks. Instead, we take sensible precautions to minimize the dangers.

That's what safer sex is all about. With a simple safeguard, like always screwing with a condom, we can easily and drastically reduce our risk of infection. The main priority is to protect each other against really dangerous diseases, such as HIV and, to a lesser extent, hepatitis B. In contrast to these two diseases, all other infections either cause no irreparable injury or are curable with treatment.

There's no reason to let fear and anxiety ruin our sense of sexual adventure and enjoyment. By adopting safer sex, we can protect ourselves, and our partners, and still have plenty of raunchy, ravishing and rapturous fun.

Preventable Diseases and Conditions
Cancers

AIDS

AIDS stands for Acquired Immune Deficiency Syndrome. It's not one disease, but a collection of over 20 different life-threatening illnesses; these include certain forms of meningitis, pneumonia, tuberculosis, herpes, cancer, dementia, candidiasis, retinitis and severe gastroenteritis. These diseases develop because the body's natural defence against infection, the immune system, gets damaged. Because it is damaged, the immune system can't fight off certain kinds of disease that our bodies can normally destroy.

The prime cause of AIDS-related immune deficiency is infection with the Human Immunodeficiency Virus (HIV). Co-factors, such as other infectious agents, stress and toxic drugs, may influence whether, or when, an infected person progresses from being healthy to developing AIDS symptoms. They may also influence the frequency and severity of AIDS diseases.

HIV damages the immune system by attacking and killing its key CD4 defender cells which coordinate our defences against disease. Over time, these cells are gradually destroyed, and the functioning of other immune defence cells is severely impaired, to the extent that the body is no longer able to defeat infections. The result is the development of the life-threatening diseases which are collectively known as AIDS. In other words, HIV is a cause and AIDS is a consequence. No one dies directly from HIV (except in the case of HIV brain disease). They die from the diseases that HIV allows to flourish.

The two main ways of acquiring HIV are sharing needles to inject drugs, and fucking without a condom. All other sexual acts, such as cock-sucking, arse-licking and finger-fucking, carry an almost negligible risk of transmitting HIV by comparison to the danger of unprotected screwing. When first infected with HIV, most people experience no symptoms of ill-health. Others have a flu-like reaction; with a temperature, body ache and fatigue. These soon pass. HIV is a very slow-acting virus. It takes an average of 10 years from the moment of getting HIV for a person to develop AIDS diseases; although some people get sick within six months, others take several years to develop illness, and some may never get ill. Throughout the incubation period, most people with HIV stay healthy, but infectious, with no outward signs of disease. It appears that a healthy lifestyle and a positive mental attitude may be two of the reasons why some people stay well longer than others. A further reason might be that they were only exposed to low doses or weak strains of HIV – which is why it is important for men with the virus to practise safer sex and avoid additional exposure. Genetic factors may also influence the rate of progression of HIV disease.

Usually it is only many years later after the date of infection, following often prolonged good health, that AIDS symptoms may begin to appear. These symptoms are signs of HIV and the various specific AIDS diseases that arise as a result of severe immune deficiency. Typically, the symptoms include two or more of the following:

- Profound and long-lasting exhaustion.
- Indefinitely swollen glands in the neck, arm-pits and groin.
- Unexplained weight loss of over 10%.
- Persistent fevers or drenching night sweats.
- Thick white spots on the tongue, gums or throat.
- Frequent diarrhoea or bloody shit.
- Unusual purple or brown skin lesions or discolorations.
- Prolonged loss of appetite or nausea.
- Recurrent and aggressive herpes, shingles or dermatitis.
- Severe and worsening headaches, dizziness, seizures or memory loss.
- Longterm shortness of breath or dry cough.

Warning: these symptoms can also be signs of common, harmless illnesses which have nothing to do with AIDS. So don't panic at the first sign of exhaustion, headache or swollen glands. People with HIV may experience persistently enlarged glands prior to developing AIDS but may remain in fairly good health for long periods.

HIV is not curable. Once people develop AIDS, most die within five years, although some survive longer. Anti-HIV drugs, such as AZT, can reduce the incidence and severity of AIDS illnesses for about a year, but they sometimes have damaging side effects. Some people believe these toxic drugs do more harm than good. Many of the specific diseases which arise as a result of HIV infection and immune deficiency can be increasingly controlled. The death rate from the AIDS pneumonia, 'PCP', has fallen dramatically with the use of aerosol pentamidine and Septrin as preventative therapies, although these too may have toxic consequences. Holistic therapies – including high-nutrition diets, vitamin supplements, meditation, visualization, acupuncture, homoeopathy, and stress reduction – can also be effective in extending people's survival time and improving the quality of their lives.

Amoebiasis and other gut infections

Amoebiasis, giardiasis, and other gut infections, such as salmonella, are caused variously by microscopic parasites or bacteria. These infections can be passed from person to person by any sexual activity which allows infected arse juices or shit to enter the mouth. Infection most commonly results from licking arse. However, it can also, very occasionally, be transmitted indirectly in two other ways. First, by finger-fucking a guy, then caressing his body and subsequently kissing the caressed areas. Second, by touching your dick, or a condom, after it has been up another guy's butt and later inadvertently putting your finger in your mouth.

The symptoms appear 1-3 weeks after infection. Depending on the particular parasitic or bacterial infection involved, these symptoms can include stomach pain, fever, nausea, vomiting, diarrhoea, tiredness, smelly farts, and mucus and blood in shit. Sometimes, prolonged infection prevents the effective absorption of food, causing malnutrition and weight loss. Gut infections are treated with antibiotics.

Cancers

Cancer is not a sexually-transmitted disease. However, there are four types of cancer which affect the area around our dicks and arses – cancer of the prostate, testicles, penis and rectum. These cancers can diminish our ability to have good sex, and may even put our lives at risk. Although cancer is not preventable in the same sense that sexually-transmitted diseases are, swift recognition and treatment usually ensures a total cure.

Prostate cancer affects the prostate gland, which nestles behind the pubic bone and against the walls of the arse. Slow-growing, the cancer causes the gland to enlarge gradually. This constricts the flow of piss from the bladder, producing difficulty or slowness in pissing. But these symptoms are also common in non-cancerous prostatitis and other relatively minor infections. Prostate cancer is normally only found in men over 50. It is detected by a doctor inserting his finger inside the arse and feeling the gland for signs of enlargement. Treatment options include irradiation, hormone therapy and surgical removal.

Testicular cancer attacks the testicles causing lumps, hardness and sometimes a dull ache. It's a good idea to feel your balls regularly and check for any of these signs. Those most at risk are men aged 20-40. With early diagnosis, nearly all cases of testicular cancer are curable by means of drug therapy or surgical removal. This does not affect a

Preventable Diseases and Conditions — Safer Sexy

man's ability to get an erection or to have enjoyable sex.

Penile cancer, which is found on the penis, variously causes abnormal growths, skin discoloration, and spots that will not heal. For guys who are uncircumsized it may also cause irritation under the foreskin. This form of cancer is very rare and is usually found only in older men. Most cases appear to be linked to poor dick hygiene over a long period. Uncut guys who do not thoroughly wash under their foreskins every day are vulnerable in later life. Chemotherapy and radiotherapy can cure penile cancer if it is detected at an early stage.

Anal and rectal cancer affect the opening of the arsehole (the anus) and the inside of the arse (the rectum). The signs are variable but can include bloody shit, stomach pain, weight loss, exhaustion, changes in bowel habits, and lumps or hardening on the outside of the arse or in the lining of the rectum. Among the various causes of anal and rectal cancer there may be a connection with genital warts in the arse. Treatment involves radiation or surgery to remove the cancerous lesions.

Chancroid

Chancroid is a bacterial disease contracted during unprotected penetrative sex. Sores appear on the dick or arse 3-6 days after infection. These can develop into painful ulcers. Soon afterwards, the glands in the groin may become swollen, hard and sore. Sometimes, they abscess and discharge pus. Chancroid can be cleared up with a course of antibiotics.

Chlamydia

Chlamydia is a very common group of bacteria which are passed on mainly by fucking, and only very rarely by cock-sucking or arse-licking.

The first signs of chlamydia appear 1-6 weeks after infection. Many infected men have no symptoms although they remain infectious and can still pass on the bacteria. Those who do have symptoms experience an abnormal whitish-yellow discharge from the dick, arse or throat. They may also have pain when pissing and an urge to piss more frequently. If untreated, the infection can spread from the cock to the prostate gland, testicles and other parts of the body. Antibiotics kill off the bacteria.

Crabs

'Crabs', or pubic lice, are tiny brown crab-like insects. They are transferred from one person to another mainly by naked body contact, such as sleeping next to an infected person or having sex with them. Less commonly, they can be caught from infested towels, sheets and clothes.

Crabs live mostly in the warm moist pubic hair around the dick, balls and arse. They cling to the skin and suck blood. This causes intense itching. Another sign is the appearance of tiny whitish-brown eggs laid on the shaft of the pubic hairs.

Crabs are a discomfort, but they cause no real harm. They and their eggs are killed by applying a special lotion over the body from the neck down which is left on for 24 hours. All clothes, sheets and towels must be washed in hot water or thoroughly ironed. Partners should be treated simultaneously to prevent reinfection.

Cystitis

Cystitis is relatively rare in men. It's a bacterial bladder infection that is very occasionally picked up when screwing arse without a condom. Germs enter the dick-hole and spread to the bladder. With cystitis you have the urge to piss frequently. Although feeling that you are about to burst, you will often only be able to piss a little. When you do piss, it causes a scalding pain and your piss may be cloudy or bloody.

Cystitis is treated with antibiotics. Left untreated, it can spread and damage the kidneys.

Glandular fever

Glandular fever is also known as 'mono', which is short for its scientific name, mononucleosis. It is a viral infection transmitted via bodily fluids, including spit and the microscopic droplets of water we exhale. This means glandular fever can be transmitted by close personal contact of a non-sexual nature, as well as from kissing and sex. It is highly infectious. Although not a serious disease, glandular fever is sometimes disabling. It can result in a high temperature, swollen glands, sore throat, extreme tiredness and body aches.

There is no treatment for glandular fever, apart from rest. Normally it clears up by itself after about four weeks, but a minority of people suffer mild symptoms for several months.

Gonorrhoea

Gonorrhoea, often nicknamed 'the clap', is caused by a bacterium. It can be passed between men by licking arse and, most often, by sucking cock and by screwing without a condom. Sometimes there are no symptoms or they are too mild to be apparent, particularly with gonorrhoea in the arse. When noticeable symptoms do appear, it is usually 2-10 days after infection. They can include a white or yellowish pus discharge from the dick, and a burning sensation when pissing or cumming. In the arse, there may be a yellowish discharge, mild diarrhoea, itching and pain when shitting. Infection via the mouth can result in a sore throat and, occasionally, a cough.

Gonorrhoea is treatable with antibiotics. Left untreated, infection can spread to the prostate gland and testicles which may lead to infertility. It can also spread to the rest of the body causing inflammation of the joints and septicaemia which can, in rare cases, be fatal.

Gut infections

See the section above on Amoebiasis.

Hepatitis

Hepatitis is a viral infection which causes inflammation of the liver. There are three main types: A, B and C. Although they all have similar symptoms, they are caught in different ways and have different consequences for longterm health.

Hepatitis A is found in shit. It is acquired by getting shit in the mouth. This can happen through contaminated food or water, or through sex. Butt-licking is very risky. Even just tonguing the outside of the arse-hole can be dangerous – more so if your partner hasn't showered since he last shitted. Screwing or fingering a guy's arse can also transmit hepatitis A. If you've been fingering someone, or you get shit on your fingers when taking off a condom, it's quite easy later on to touch your mouth and swallow the virus unawares. To reduce the risk, get your partner to shower thoroughly if you want to lick the outside of his arse-hole; use a latex barrier if you plan to stick your tongue inside his butt; wash your hands if you have touched anything that may have had shit on it.

The symptoms of hepatitis A appear 2-6 weeks after infection. These can include headache, fever, loss of appetite (particularly for fatty foods and alcohol), nausea, vomiting, lethargy, and muscle and joint pains. A little later, the eye-balls and skin may go yellow (jaundice). Piss can turn dark brown and shit near-white. The liver, which is just below the stomach on the left, may

Preventable Diseases and Conditions
Non-specific urethritis and proctitis

become tender. Of course, not everyone with hepatitis A has such pronounced symptoms. In some the symptoms are unremarkable. The only treatment for hepatitis A is plenty of rest, a low-protein and high-carbohydrate diet, and the avoidance of fat and alcohol. The illness clears up by itself within 1-3 months and causes no lasting damage.

Men who regularly lick the arses of lots of different partners are strongly advised to protect themselves by getting vaccinated against hepatitis A.

Hepatitis B can be transmitted by blood, serum, cum, spit, piss and shit. This means that it is much more infectious than hepatitis A, or HIV. Safer sex will not necessarily protect you. Unlike HIV, you can get hepatitis B from deep kissing. Compared to HIV, it is much easier to contract hepatitis B from cock-sucking, arse-licking, ingesting shit or getting another guy's piss inside you. Like HIV, of course, hepatitis B can also be acquired from fucking without a condom, jerking off where cum gets into open wounds, fisting which exchanges blood, swopping sex toys which enter the body, and sharing needles during injecting drug use.

While a majority of people get over hepatitis B and cease to be infectious, about 10% remain longterm virus carriers who are able to infect others for many years. Hepatitis B has a long incubation period of 1-6 months. During this time, a person is infectious but the infection may not be obvious nor easily detectable. When symptoms eventually do manifest, they are usually similar to those of hepatitis A. Sometimes, however, they are barely noticeable or may be mistaken for flu. Most people with hepatitis B remain ill for 1-2 months, normally without requiring hospitalization. A small proportion suffer many months of debilitating illness. In extreme cases, hepatitis B can lead to liver cirrhosis and cancer, and possibly death.

As well as lots of rest and the avoidance of alcohol, the main treatment for hepatitis B is alpha interferon injections.

Hepatitis B is totally preventable through a vaccination, which gives protection over several years. Since a significant number of gay men are infectious carriers, getting a hepatitis B jab is strongly recommended.

Hepatitis C is also known as 'non-A, non-B hepatitis'. While it produces symptoms like those of hepatitis A and B, neither of these other viruses are detectable in people with hepatitis C. Avoiding the risky behaviour that causes hepatitis A and B also protects you against hepatitis C.

The incubation period, duration and treatment of hepatitis C mirrors that of hepatitis A. It can also occasionally lead to chronic liver disease and cancer.

Herpes

There are two forms of herpes. Cold sores are caused by the Herpes Simplex Virus type 1 (HSV1). Cold sores appear on, or around, the lips or nose. Genital herpes is caused by the related Herpes Simplex Virus type 2 (HSV2). It is found in, or near, the dick or arse. Of the two varieties, HSV2 is the more severe and painful infection. The two viruses are interchangeable. Cold sores on the mouth can be spread to the cock and arse, and genital herpes can be spread to the mouth.

Cold sores and genital herpes are both usually characterized by small blisters filled with a clear liquid which later turns to a yellow pus. These blisters variously tingle, sting and itch. When they burst it can be excruciatingly painful. They then develop into red ulcers which scab over and heal after 1-3 weeks. Genital herpes inside the dick-hole causes agonizing pain when pissing or cumming. In the arse, it results in a burning sensation, especially during shitting. Some people who get cold sores and genital herpes have recurrent attacks every few months, particularly when they are feeling stressed, tired or sick. These attacks can also be triggered by exposure to ultra violet light, as occurs during prolonged sun-bathing. Attacks often become less frequent and less severe over time.

Both forms of herpes can be transferred from one person to another by touch. Handling an infected dick and then touching your lip or arse, could transmit the virus. However, it is most often passed on by fucking without a rubber, and sometimes by kissing, sucking dick, licking or fingering arse and sharing sex toys.

Shortly before the herpes blisters appear, and later while they are visible, a person is highly infectious. Afterwards, when they crust over, the virus becomes dormant and non-contagious. Although an infected man will carry the virus for the rest of his life, the risk of him passing it on once the herpes sores have healed and disappeared is very small. He can resume sexual relations.

At the first signs of either type of herpes it is very important to avoid all sexual activities which involve the affected area coming into contact with your partner's body. No cock-sucking or kissing, for example, when you have cold sores on your mouth. No rubbing cocks together when he has ulcers on his dick. While you're in the infectious period, avoid sharing soap or towels, and always wash your hands thoroughly before touching another guy, especially on the mouth, arse or dick.

There is no cure for either type of herpes. Anti-viral treatments can, however, ease the pain and shorten the duration of an outbreak. People who suffer from recurrent herpes can be given suppressant therapies which help to prevent attacks and reduce the risk of infecting a partner.

HIV

See the section above on AIDS.

Molluscum contagiosum

Molluscum contagiosum is caused by a virus which can be spread by any form of body contact with the infection, including sucking, licking and fucking. It results in small white pearl-like growths. These are painless and can appear anywhere on the skin. In sexually-transmitted molluscum contagiosum, they usually appear on the inside or the outside of the cock or arse. After 6-10 weeks, the infection often disappears spontaneously. Persistent cases can be treated with growth-destroying chemicals, and by burning or freezing.

Non-specific urethritis and proctitis

Non-specific urethritis (NSU) is also referred to as non-gonococcal urethritis (NGU). It's an infection of the urethra, or dick-hole, through which we piss and cum. Doctors call NSU 'non-specific', because it is often not possible to identify the infectious organism responsible. Some cases are caused by chlamydia. Others appear to occur spontaneously, for no apparent reason, without any sexual contact. But mostly you get it from fucking without a condom. Very occasionally, you can get it if a guy with NSU in his mouth sucks your cock, or if you suck a guy with an infected dick.

NSU can be present without any symptoms. If symptoms do appear it is normally 1-3 weeks after infection. Signs can include a sharp, cutting pain when pissing or having sex, and a white or yellow discharge from the cock which tends to be most noticeable when you get up in the morning. This discharge may leave stains on your underwear or sheets. Sometimes, the glands in your groin can become inflamed and tender.

Non-specific proctitis (NSP) is the same as

Preventable Diseases and Conditions — Safer Sexy

NSU, only it is found in the arse. It is nearly always acquired through screwing without a rubber. NSP is accompanied by an off-white discharge from the butt, which may cause slight itching or discomfort.

Both NSP and NSU can be cured successfully with antibiotics.

Prostatitis

Prostatitis is an infection of the prostate gland. It can sometimes be contracted from bacteria entering the dick-hole during unsafe screwing. Symptoms can include swelling of the prostate gland, occasional blood in piss and cum, fever, an ache behind the base of the dick, and pain during pissing or cumming. Antibiotics will clear up the infection but recurrences are common and long courses of treatment may be necessary.

Scabies

Scabies is caused by a tiny parasitic mite that lives just under the surface of the skin – most often around the arse, groin, ankles, waist, wrists, arm-pits and between the toes and fingers. It causes a red, bumpy and extremely itchy rash in the affected areas. Scabies can be spread by any form of skin-to-skin contact. It can also be acquired from infested clothes, towels and sheets.

Treatment consists of painting the whole body, except the head, with a chemical lotion that is left on for 24 hours; plus washing all bedding, clothing and towelling in the hottest cycle of the washing machine. Even after successful treatment itching may continue for up to two weeks.

Syphilis

Syphilis is a very serious bacterial disease transmitted overwhelmingly through fucking arse without a condom, and less commonly through sucking dick and butt-licking. The symptoms develop in three stages:

First, in the 1-10 weeks after infection, a small painless sore or hardened lump appears near the point where the bacteria entered the body – this could be the cock, arse or mouth. Second, 2-6 months later, the infected person experiences a rash on the body and a flu-like illness involving fever, headache and a sore throat. The symptoms during these first two stages may sometimes be mild and difficult to spot. Third, if left untreated, many years later the infection can cause strokes, paralysis, blindness, brain damage and heart attacks.

Syphilis is detectable via a blood test and is completely curable with antibiotics, causing no permanent harm – if it's treated early.

Trichomoniasis

Trichomoniasis, commonly known as 'trich', is due to a small protozoa that can infect the arse and dick during unprotected fucking. The signs are discomfort when pissing, especially first thing in the morning, and a thin clear or yellow-green discharge which may be frothy in appearance. Trich often produces no noticeable symptoms. However, carriers remain infectious. Treatment is with antibiotics.

Warts

Warts are abnormal skin growths caused by the human papilloma virus (HPV). Related forms of this virus produce warts on the genitals and hands. Indeed, it's possible to transfer warts from your hand to your arse when you finger-fuck yourself, or from another guy's hand to your cock when he jerks you off. Although this form of transmission is relatively rare, to be safe it is worthwhile getting hand warts treated promptly.

Genital warts are found on the outside, or inside, of the dick and arse. Usually white or pink, they come in different shapes and sizes: flat and smooth, rough and bumpy, small and isolated, and large cauliflower-like clusters. They periodically cause itching or pain, particularly if you get them inside your dick-hole or up your arse. If this happens, it can cause severe discomfort and sometimes bleeding when you piss, shit, screw and cum. Bleeding from warts on the dick or in the arse can increase the chance of giving or getting HIV. Warts can also tear condoms. Get them treated fast.

It takes an average of three months after the date of infection for genital warts to become visible, although they can appear as soon as two weeks, or as long as a year, after the virus is contracted. During this invisible latent period, a person can nevertheless be infectious. Occasionally, the wart virus may be present, but never develop into noticeable skin growths. However, the carrier can still pass the virus on to others.

Genital warts are transmitted by touch during sex. This means that any sexual act involving contact with a wart infection can potentially transfer the virus. While screwing without a rubber is by far the most risky activity, sucking an infected dick or licking an infected arse also carries some risk of developing genital-type warts on, or in, the mouth. Guys with genital warts therefore need to keep their infected body parts out of reach of other men until they are cured. Without treatment, warts multiply and spread. One can become dozens. There is also a possibilty that untreated genital warts may be linked to the subsequent development of cancer of the dick or arse.

Treatment options include painting the warts with killer chemicals, freezing them with liquid nitrogen, burning them with acid or lasers or, as a last resort, surgical removal.

The ABC of prevention

A Choose safer sex: if you fuck, use a condom.
B Get vaccinated against hepatitis A and B.
C Cover sores, cuts and warts.
D Avoid contact with cold sores.
E Practise good body hygiene.
F Have a regular check-up at an STD clinic.
G Get medical advice if you have any sign of infection, such as a rash, sore, wart, lump, swelling, discharge, itching, or bloody piss or shit.

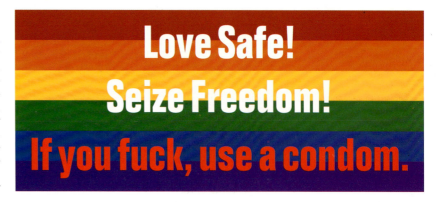

Love Safe! Seize Freedom! If you fuck, use a condom.